HAPPY  YOU!

YOUR ROADMAP TO THE GOOD LIFE

Dr. Wendy Schauer, D.C.
Foreword by, Kevin Hogan, PsyD

Copyright 2024

Abundant Fitness Publishing

All Rights Reserved

ISBN: 979-8-9889786-2-6

PRAISE FOR HAPPY NEW YOU!

"Dr. Wendy Schauer's 'Happy New You' stands out for its holistic approach to wellness, making complex concepts easy to understand and apply. This book offers a comprehensive yet straightforward roadmap for transforming your health and happiness. It's a blueprint for a healthier, happier life that anyone can follow."

Gabby Reece
Podcast Host, Speaker, Author, Athlete

What an incredible book! Dr. Wendy gives you a crash course on EVERYTHING you need to know to go from where you are now to where you want to be! Change is possible. Happiness is possible. Abundance (in every area of your life!) is possible. Release any preconceived notions you may have about "self-help" or "personal development." This book will transform your life if you let it!!!

Brent Webb
Mind Power Expert
Santa Monica, CA
www.BrentWebb.com

Dr. Wendy possesses a unique talent for maintaining absolute focus in her teachings, ensuring every word counts with no fluff in sight. She masterfully conveys what most authors take many more words to express, utilizing only about 10% of the typical word count. In "Happy New You!", she distills the essence of starting a healthy lifestyle into concise, powerful lessons. This efficiency allows you to quickly grasp the necessary knowledge, freeing up more time for you to actively engage with the essential action steps required for your transformation.

Tom Broadwell
Author of 'Lazy F*cks Don't Live to 100'

Most self-help books focus on one particular topic: diet, positive thinking, etc. "Happy New You!" can be considered your primer for living your best life in just one easy-to-read book in a step-by-step, non-overwhelming fashion. If you truly want to change your life or even just refresh it, this is the only book you will need.

Fred Pescatore, MD, MPH
Best-Selling author of
'The Hamptons Diet' & 'The A-List Diet'

This is a great book. If you apply the wisdom in it, you are going to be amazed!

Matt Furey
Psycho-Cybernetics.com
Author of 'One Breath at a Time'

Happy New You by Dr. Wendy Schauer is like the "owner's manual for life" that we all need... but don't get. This book guides the reader to get the most out of our journey by exploring ways to create a stellar life from every angle, from developing physical, mental, emotional, and spiritual health to strengthening the qualities of our own internal and external environment. An ambitious book that seems to leave no stone unturned in the human experience, this is the book for anyone who wants to pursue the effort to become the best version of themselves.

D.J. Vanas,
Author of 'The Warrior Within' and Host of the PBS Special
'Discovering Your Warrior Spirit'

Dr. Wendy's "Happy New You!" brilliantly encapsulates the essence of self-improvement and life mastery. Each of the 52 steps is a stepping stone to greater success, learning, and personal fulfillment. For those committed to creating a meaningful and impactful life, this book is your guide to the top.

Gary Ryan Blair - The GoalsGuy!
www.100DayChallenge.com

Ready for a "Happy New You"? Dr. Wendy shares 52 ways to create a better you and a better life. My suggestion is to read one chapter per week, focus on that one idea of a Happy New You, and apply it to your life. Guaranteed, you will be a very different person in just a few weeks. Then, in one year, you will be shocked at how amazing your life is. Buy a copy for a friend, spouse, or co-worker and do this together.

Croix Sather
Author, Speaker, & World Record Holder

"Dr. Wendy Schauer uses research and experience to help move the reader in practical and easy-to-understand ways towards sustainable positive change."

Shawn Achor
NYTimes bestselling author of
'Big Potential' and 'The Happiness Advantage'

DISCLAIMER

"Happy New You!" is presented as a compilation of thoughts, tools, and experiences designed to inspire personal growth and happiness. The content, a result of extensive research and collaboration with experts, is intended for informational purposes only. While the book aims to serve as a guiding light on your personal journey, it's crucial to understand that its effectiveness relies on your willingness to absorb, reflect, and act on its teachings responsibly.

The perspectives and suggestions within this book are rooted in personal experiences and collective wisdom. They are not intended to diagnose, treat, or offer any form of medical, financial, or legal advice. The transformative power and responsibility to effect change lie firmly within you, and your path will be sculpted by your unique experiences, challenges, and aspirations. If you are facing challenges or situations in these areas—particularly concerning mental health—it is essential to consult with licensed professionals who can provide specialized guidance tailored to your needs.

This book provides information "as is" without any guarantees or warranties, express or implied. Despite every effort to ensure accuracy and completeness, the author and publisher are not responsible for any errors, omissions, or outcomes resulting from the use of this information. The views and opinions expressed are those of the author(s) and do not necessarily reflect official policies or positions of any other agency, organization, or company. These views are not intended to malign any religion, ethnic group, club, organization, company, or individual.

By reading "Happy New You!", you acknowledge that the author and publisher are not providing specific professional advice. Any liability or responsibility for any loss, damage, injury, claim, or any adverse effect arising from the application of the information in this book is expressly disclaimed.

The strategies, opinions, and advice presented are based on the author's experiences and research and may not necessarily apply universally. This book is not affiliated with or endorsed by any organization or professional body.

Embark on this transformative journey with enthusiasm and caution. Remember, the choices you make and the outcomes that unfold are a reflection of your actions and decisions. Proceed with wisdom and due consultation with relevant experts, especially in matters of health, finance, legal issues, or personal well-being. May your journey through these pages be filled with enlightenment, resilience, and joy.

DEDICATION

This book is dedicated to all of you who have touched my life with warmth and inspiration; I am profoundly grateful. It is also dedicated to those who brought challenges and tests. Thank you for helping mold my resilience and perspective. Each of you, whether through love or lessons, has illuminated the path to this "Happy New You!" This book celebrates both our shared and unique journeys.

ACKNOWLEDGMENT

I first would like to thank all of the people who have come to see me for chiropractic care. I have learned so much from you. Without you, this book wouldn't have happened.

I would like to acknowledge my husband, Gary, who has been my biggest supporter, cheerleader, and sounding board. He has been by my side since the beginning and has believed in me in times when I didn't believe in myself. Thank you, Gary, and I love you.

Kevin Hogan has been a mentor and dear friend for years. He was a voice of reason when I had to make a huge life decision. In my panic and depression, he was there for me, helping me tease out the options to make a decision that had an 85% chance of going right. He didn't placate me and say everything was going to be okay, but he talked through the options and what possibly could go right or wrong. It ended up being great, and I am eternally grateful for you taking my call from a crying, stressed-out friend. Thank you, Kevin, for being in my life.

Thank you to Pavel Tsatsouline, founder of StrongFirst. He introduced me to kettlebells in the early 2000s when my back was bad, I was living in a back support, and I was on the verge of losing my career. He gave me guidance and support to start using kettlebells to strengthen my core and back. He was a lifesaver, and I was able to continue my work as a chiropractor. Pavel is a dear friend, and I am eternally grateful.

Thank you to Mark Edgar Stephens, who has been a big inspiration in my life. In Mark's book, "Who Are You Choosing To Be?" he has his readers ask, "What is the blessing?" when negative life events take over. I don't think he realizes how often I use that phrase, even when I don't want to. It helps me to shift my perspective and find the positive even in a very negative situation. Thank you, Mark, for all of the work we did together.

I am extremely fortunate that I have an amazing family and a second family that supports me through all of my endeavors. My parents, Ron and Patricia, my brother Scott and his wife Leslie, and my in-laws, Connie and Michael, have all been behind me supporting me along the way. Thank you, and I love you all.

APPRECIATION

A very special thank you and outpouring of appreciation to these wonderful people that I have been beyond blessed to have in my life.

DiAnne Busse, Kelsey Cornejo, Klaudia Conradt, Travis Jacobsen, Jennifer Lehmann, Angi Reeves, Jesse Reeves, Angelina Ryan, Mark J. Ryan, Cheri Sanderson, Dave Sloan, Heather Sloan, Beth Watkins, George Zaharoff, and Jane Robinson

FOREWORD

The Black Swans Leave

The Black Swan is a representation of dramatic negative events. Someone gets hurt badly, and another dies. There's a divorce, a lost job, a heart-stopping diagnosis.

Before someone moves on a path toward an often elusive happiness, it's worth knowing that these Black Swan occurrences are not completely random. Sometimes, people have more responsibilities and are more responsible to more people than others. They have more exposure to negative events than others.

That said, just because exposure to something doesn't mean a worst-case scenario in every instance is an important notion. Just because it happened last time doesn't mean it will happen again. Pessimism is known to reduce a satisfying life.

What is pessimism anyway? It's really about how you explain your negative life experiences to yourself and the world. Have you ever noticed how people who don't accept responsibility blame everyone but themselves? Well...yeah...they often are happier than other people. I'm not going to go so far as to ask you to point fingers when something goes wrong. That's ridiculous. Blame is for spoiled children. "Who's to blame?"

You read that online, and you hear people ask that question. Or maybe you hear, "It's THEIR fault." It's not the person you want to be, but you want the result of being happier and having a more satisfying life. I'm going to ask you to make a shift on all of this. "I'm not going to let this happen again." That's one new mantra for the year of living a better life.

The best psychological research shows that it is first the fact that some people blame themselves instead of events when things go wrong. That is dangerous. Blame is often a complete blackening of a clean sheet of paper, like turning off all the lights on a cloudy night. It gets dark fast, and so can life when people walk around with self-blame. Understand when you make a mistake, it's a good thing to say, "I screwed up on that ONE." Or perhaps, "I'm not going to let that mistake happen again."

The next piece of the pessimism triangle is that bad things always have happened to you and always will. (Permanence) "This sh*& always happens to me." And a lot of sh*& does happen to you, sometimes. And sometimes, you really do have more than most people. That is part of the human experience. It's certainly not "fair," but it's important to know that yesterday's disaster might have been the last king-sized disaster for quite a while. And sometimes you get 5 in a month. But they don't have to last forever, nor do they always have to happen to you.

As bad stuff happens in life, create a rational distance from it. Certainly, solve the problems that call the black swans, remembering that most really are random.

You and I don't know where it will flood tomorrow. We don't know where the fires will start. We can't know who will get a bad diagnosis. Nor do we know if it will come to its worst case.

Next time there is a goofball in line at Costco or a noisy nut on the street, instead of letting the emotions you have experienced in the past consume you and using up your Life Units on being angry, fearful, etc., simply shake your head and say, "Oh my...life is interesting."

Change your thinking and stop commenting or even paying attention to the madness of other human beings.

After you have begun to watch some of the problems and disasters of life slowly move away from you, recognize that simply watching them move slowly out of your life or away from your pain buttons can be very freeing. It's not going to be easy to do this. It is an exercise of shifting how you perceive lots of things.

It might not hurt to watch for that moment when something GOOD actually happens to you, and you literally say, in that moment, "And it's true that lots of good things happen in my life." Because I bet they do. There might be as much bad or even worse, but LOTS of GOOD things happen in life. This is not some flimsy "affirmation" from a ridiculous self-help book. Instead, it is a way of cutting out a positive aspect of life and recognizing when it does happen.

Before Dr. Schauer takes the stage in this most significant book, I want you to avoid affirmations in general. "I feel terrific," when you don't, does you no good.

Instead, tell yourself, "I feel terrific," in the moment you actually do so, your brain begins a library of GOOD life moments.

Life is difficult. Life is also typically worth being here for tomorrow and the next day.

Now, I will introduce you to one of my favorite people on the planet. A truly caring and compassionate human being, Dr. Wendy Schauer.

Kevin Hogan
Minneapolis
2024

CONTENTS

PREFACE 1

INTRODUCTION 3

CHAPTER 1: The Power Of Being Willing To Learn 8

CHAPTER 2: Embrace The Power Of Being Coachable 12

CHAPTER 3: Breathe – Harnessing The Power Of Deep Diaphragmatic Breathing 17

CHAPTER 4: Hydration – Quenching Your Body's Thirst For Vitality 21

CHAPTER 5: Embracing The Power Of Restful Sleep 26

CHAPTER 6: Mindful Consumption – Gi/Go 31

CHAPTER 7: The Power Of Alkalizing Foods – Nourishing Your Body's Balance 36

CHAPTER 8: Embrace The Power Of Daily Movement 41

CHAPTER 9: Get Things Moving – Nurturing Regular Bowel Health 46

CHAPTER 10: The Essential Vitamins You Need 51

CHAPTER 11: Unleash The Power Of Reading – Ignite Your Path To Success 56

CHAPTER 12: Stretching Beyond Limits – Expanding Body And Mind 60

CHAPTER 13: Embrace The Power Of Walking – Small Steps, Big Impact 65

CHAPTER 14: Embrace The Sun 72

CHAPTER 15: Get Grounded – Reconnecting With The Earth's Energy 77

CHAPTER 16: Mastering The Basics – Building A Strong Foundation For Success 81

CHAPTER 17: Exercise – The Power Of Starting Simple 85

CHAPTER 18: Financial Success On $7 A Day - Unleashing The 8th Wonder Of The World 90

CHAPTER 19: The Richest Man In Babylon - Building Wealth And Embracing Financial Freedom 95

CHAPTER 20: The Power Of Massage For Your Happy New You 99

CHAPTER 21: Discovering The Power Of Chiropractic Care 104

CHAPTER 22: Get Unplugged - Embrace Nature And Disconnect For Inner Peace 108

CHAPTER 23: The Ripple Effect Of Kindness - Spreading Joy One Act At A Time 112

CHAPTER 24: The Liberating Power Of Forgiveness - Embrace The Gift Of Release 116

CHAPTER 25: The Magic Of Thank You Cards - Spreading More Gratitude And Joy 120

CHAPTER 26: Always Move Forward—Embrace Progression 124

CHAPTER 27: Detoxify Your Life—Embrace A Healthier And Happier You 131

CHAPTER 28: Embrace The Minimalist Lifestyle —Discover The Freedom Of Letting Go 136

CHAPTER 29: Spend More Time With Family And Friends—The Power Of Connection 141

CHAPTER 30: Fish Or Cut Bait—Embrace The Power Of Taking Action 145

CHAPTER 31: Increase Your Likability Factor For A Happier Life 149

CHAPTER 32: The Power Of Managing Expectations For A Happy New Life 153

CHAPTER 33: The Healing Power Of Laughter—Embrace The Joyful Side Of Life 158

CHAPTER 34: The Art Of Gratitude—Embrace The Power Of Maybe Yes, Maybe No 162

CHAPTER 35: The Power Of Relaxation—Embrace The Art Of Letting Go 167

CHAPTER 36: Sitting Is The New Smoking—Reclaim Your Health And Vitality 172

CHAPTER 37: Hang Your Way To A Healthier Spine And Stronger Grip 177

CHAPTER 38: Unleashing Your Creative Potential—Embrace The Power Of Imagination 182

CHAPTER 39: Cultivating Resilience—Bouncing Back Stronger Than Ever.....190

CHAPTER 40: Nurturing Self-Compassion—Embrace Your Imperfections.....195

CHAPTER 41: Make Your Bed—A Small Act With Great Impact 200

CHAPTER 42: Achieving Gold With Visualization 204

CHAPTER 43: Embracing Failure—The Courage To Continue....................... 210

CHAPTER 44: Transforming Fear Into Power— Breaking Through Limiting Beliefs 214

CHAPTER 45: The Power Of Mentorship And Continuous Learning...............218

CHAPTER 46: Overcoming Procrastination And Taking Action With The 5 Second Rule 223

CHAPTER 47: Cultivating Patience—Trusting The Process Of Growth......... 228

CHAPTER 48: Embracing Change—Thriving In Times Of Transition 233

CHAPTER 49: The Power Of Empathy— Connecting With Others' Hearts.....239

CHAPTER 50: Track Your Progress—Celebrating Your Wins And Sustaining Your Happy New You Journey 245

CHAPTER 51: The Power Of Ownership—Embrace Your Destiny With 100% Responsibility.. 250

CHAPTER 52: Celebrating Your Happy New You—Reflecting On A Year Of Growth And Transformation..256

SUGGESTED READING 264
REFERENCES...265
ABOUT THE AUTHOR 277

PREFACE

As I sit here writing this from my hotel balcony, the vastness of the ocean before me, the steady rhythm of the waves crashing, becomes an echoing affirmation of life's perpetual motion. The salty breeze, interspersed with the distant cries of seagulls, is a sensory reminder of nature's capacity to heal, invigorate, and inspire.

Nature has a profound way of switching on our happiness neurotransmitters. The very act of immersing oneself in its presence- be it a forest, mountain, or, in my case, a serene beach- can catalyze a surge of positivity. Today, with every grain of sand that sifted through my fingers, I felt a renewed charge, a deeper connection to the world, and an overwhelming urge to share this sensation of joy.

However, as joyous as this moment is for me, I am deeply aware of an unsettling contrast. The World Happiness Report, which assesses global well-being, often paints a less rosy picture of the United States. Despite our nation's prosperity and advancements, we do not rank even in the top 10 of happiest nations. The U.S. tends to be between 15-19 on the scale. Such findings aren't mere statistics; they're a mirror reflecting collective emotions, an indication that a large number of individuals are battling internal storms.

Even more concerning is the data from the National Institute of Mental Health. In 2019, an astounding 19.2 million adults in the U.S. experienced at least one major depressive episode. These aren't just faceless numbers; these are fellow humans, possibly our neighbors, friends, or family members, grappling with the weight of despair.

In writing "Happy New You!", my intentions stretched beyond merely writing a book. This work is a manifestation of my deepest desires- a hope for happiness, not just for me, but for every reader, their loved ones, and the broader human family. In my three-decade career as a chiropractor, I've borne witness to the physical and emotional ailments of countless humans. While each person's story is unique, a common thread often emerges the yearning for happiness, contentment, and a break from life's relentless pressures.

Yet, here is a pivotal realization- this book, as comprehensive and heartfelt as it is, isn't an elixir or panacea. It is a stepping stone, an invitation to embark on a journey towards consistent happiness. It is a hand extended in partnership, offering insights, reflections, and strategies to navigate the often-tumultuous waters of life.

Our pursuit of happiness is often ensnared by external validations- the next big purchase, the job promotion, the idealized life presented on social media. Yet, true happiness, as I have come to discover, especially in moments like this amidst nature, is internal. It is a state of mind, a conscious choice, and a commitment to one's well-being.

With this book, I invite you to join me in redefining and rediscovering happiness. It is a journey, one that requires introspection, understanding, and action. While the path might be strewn with challenges, the destination- a state of consistent joy and fulfillment- is worth every effort.

In sharing these words, insights, and experiences, I hope "Happy New You!" serves as a beacon of hope, guiding you towards brighter days, inner peace, and the countless joys in life, in its infinite beauty, has to offer.

Warmly,
Dr. Wendy

INTRODUCTION

Picture this: 35,000 feet in the air, gazing down at the sprawling landscapes below, I embark on yet another journey - not just across states but through the tapestry of a life lived fully and fiercely. As I leave Seattle behind, heading towards Bend, Oregon, to celebrate my 58th birthday and Thanksgiving with my family, I am reminded of the incredible journey that has brought me here.

From the time I was a young girl, mistaking my family's homelessness for an extended camping trip, to the woman I am today, my life has been a mosaic of resilience, determination, and triumph. Each chapter of my story, marked by both struggle and success, has shaped my perspective and fueled a burning desire to make each day count.

In this book, I unfold the themes that have been the bedrock of my journey - resilience, hard work, and the relentless pursuit of excellence. These are not just abstract concepts; they are the lived experiences that have propelled me from a cramped, one-bedroom apartment to a life where my family, my cherished partner of 30 years, and a thriving business are my proud achievements.

But let's get real - my story is not a tale of overnight success. It's about the grind, the hustle, and the unwavering commitment to a vision. It's about working six jobs simultaneously, about turning the challenges of life into opportunities for growth. This journey, while uniquely mine, is also yours. It's a story of what happens when you refuse to give up, no matter the odds.

As you delve into these pages, you'll find not just my story but also the tools and strategies that have been my compass. This book is a guide, a mentor, and a friend, offering you the wisdom I have gathered from a lifetime of learning and overcoming.

> Like this cup, you are full of your own opinions and speculations. How can I show you Zen unless you first empty your cup?
>
> **Zen parable.**

In the gentle folds of an ancient Zen Garden, where each purposely placed stone and carefully raked sand pattern serves as a testament to mindfulness, the spirit of powerful teaching whispers through the leaves of the cherry blossoms. This teaching immortalized through a parable of a simple cup of tea, has transcended time and space to arrive here, in your hands, at the beginning of your journey with "Happy New You!"

Picture a traditional Japanese tearoom where a well-respected university professor has sought the wisdom of a renowned Zen master. The room is suffused with the subtle scent of incense, tatami mats underfoot, and the shoji screens, diffusing the light into a soft embrace. The Zen master, an embodiment of tranquility, begins the tea ceremony —a dance of grace and intention, every movement a lesson in itself.

The professor, eager to expand his intellect, watches intently, his mind racing with questions and theories. As the master pours the tea, the liquid meets the brim but does not cease its flow. It spills over, a stream of warmth overrunning the confines of ceramic edges, much to the professor's dismay. It is at this crucial juncture that the Zen master imparts a lesson profound in its simplicity: 'Like this cup, you are full of your own opinions and speculations. How can I show you Zen unless you first empty your cup?'

This moment, rich with symbolism, is where our introduction to "Happy New You!" begins. It is a poignant reminder that the cup we hold—brimming with past experiences, beliefs, and biases—must be emptied if we are to make room for the new. And what is "Happy New You!" if not a vessel for the new?

You hold in your hands a promise, a canvas of 52 weeks upon which you will paint new habits, thoughts, and actions. Each week represents a unique opportunity to lay a stone on your path of personal evolution. This is not the path of radical change but of nurturing growth, where every small step is a deliberate and defining stride toward the person you aspire to become.

Your journey through "Happy New You!" is a pilgrimage of sorts, a voyage that will challenge you to unlearn in order to learn anew. In the pages that follow, you will not find quick fixes or shortcuts; instead, you will discover the joy of gradual unfolding, the strength in vulnerability, and the peace that comes with self-acceptance.

The structure of this journey is designed to guide you gently but firmly. Each chapter, representing a week, is a blend of philosophy and action—a concept to reflect upon and a corresponding practice to weave into the fabric of your daily life. It is a methodical approach rooted in the belief that true transformation is a gradual alchemy of the soul.

As you immerse yourself in the initial chapters, you may feel the resistance of the mind, the tug of skepticism, or the weight of habitual thinking. This is the clutter of a cup too full, and it is natural. Acknowledge, don't fight, these feelings, for they are part of your current fullness. But also, invite them to leave to make way for the new insights that will soon begin to fill you.

Each subsequent week will build upon the last, creating a mosaic of change. You will explore themes of gratitude, presence, mindfulness, and resilience. You will be invited to challenge old paradigms, embrace your imperfections, and celebrate your victories, no matter how small. As the weeks unfold, so too will the layers of your being, revealing the depths of your character and the heights of your potential.

Approach every exercise, every piece of wisdom, with the openness of the cup before it overflows. Be willing to pour out the old tea, the stale remnants of past brews, in order to savor the fresh infusion of perspectives that "Happy New You!" offers. Remember, it is in the space of not knowing, of curiosity and wonder, that the most potent learning occurs. It is here, in the unburdening of the known, that change is born.

This book will challenge you to be brave, to stand at the edge of your comfort zone, and to step beyond it. It will encourage you to look inward, to confront both the shadows and the light within, and to embrace them both. It will celebrate your entire being and will serve as a mirror to reflect your true self back to you.

"Happy New You!" is your companion on this adventure, a testament to the belief that transformation is accessible to all who are willing to embark on the journey. With each chapter, each week, you will not only be moving towards a new you but also deepening the relationship with you that has always been—the essence of your being.

As you ready yourself to begin, take a deep, cleansing breath. Let it sweep through you, clearing away the dust of doubt and the cobwebs of hesitation. Hold this book before you as if it were the cup offered by the Zen master—empty, receptive, and open to being filled with golden wisdom.

Prepare to laugh, to cry, to be challenged, and to be affirmed. Prepare for moments of profound realization and quiet introspection. Prepare for the transformation that is not a dramatic unveiling but a soft, subtle awakening to the dawn of a "Happy New You."

Welcome to the beginning of your new chapter. Welcome to an adventure of becoming. Welcome, with an open heart and an empty cup, to the transformative journey that awaits.

> **THE CAPACITY TO LEARN IS A GIFT; THE ABILITY TO LEARN IS A SKILL; THE WILLINGNESS TO LEARN IS A CHOICE.**
>
> — BRIAN HERBERT

CHAPTER 1
THE POWER OF BEING WILLING TO LEARN

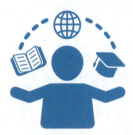

Welcome to "Happy New You!" where we explore the transformative concept of being willing to learn. I chose this as the first chapter, as the willingness to learn is the catalyst for personal and professional growth, propelling you toward a life of fulfillment, success, and continuous improvement.

In a rapidly changing world, adaptability is crucial for thriving. Being open to learning empowers you to embrace change with curiosity and navigate new situations, technologies, and challenges confidently, while those who resist learning may find themselves left behind.

Learning unlocks your full potential, propelling you forward on the path of self-discovery and growth. Seeking knowledge enriches your understanding of the world and your capabilities, paving the way to become the best version of yourself in various areas of life.

Life presents challenges and opportunities. Being willing to learn equips you with problem-solving skills, providing valuable resources to address obstacles effectively. The more you learn, the more creative and innovative your solutions become, paving the way for unprecedented achievements.

Open communication and collaboration are at the heart of successful relationships. A genuine willingness to learn from others nurtures meaningful connections. Being attentive and receptive to their experiences and perspectives enriches both your personal and professional life. Unfortunately, we are in a world right now where people immediately judge and shut down all communication with others. Now is the time to be open and willing. We can all learn from those who are different from us.

The pursuit of learning is a journey of personal development and self-discovery. Immersing yourself in various subjects leads to profound insights into your strengths, weaknesses, and aspirations, becoming the foundation for a life aligned with your passions and purpose.

In the professional realm, a commitment to learning is highly prized. Embracing learning opens doors to career advancement and increased opportunities, positioning you as an invaluable asset to any team or organization. According to Warren Buffett, "The more you learn, the more you earn."

Being willing to learn helps you to become more resilient. Viewing challenges as learning opportunities reframes setbacks as stepping stones toward growth. With a willingness to adapt and improve, you bounce back stronger, ready to face whatever comes your way.

Learning broadens horizons, exposing you to new ideas, cultures, and ways of thinking. Embracing different perspectives fosters open-mindedness and empathy. Learning becomes a journey of understanding and celebrating the rich tapestry of humanity.

Embrace the power of being willing to learn. It is a mindset that transforms challenges into opportunities and obstacles into advantages. The willingness to learn empowers you to navigate through life's twists and turns, creating a future of endless possibilities.

In the chapters ahead, we will explore strategies to cultivate a hunger for knowledge and wisdom. Get ready to unleash your true potential and embrace the power of being willing to learn, for within it lies the key to a "Happy New You!"

> **THE ONLY TRUE WISDOM IS IN KNOWING YOU KNOW NOTHING.**
>
> — SOCRATES

CHAPTER 2
EMBRACE THE POWER OF BEING COACHABLE

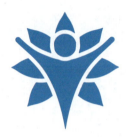

In the journey towards personal and professional growth, we encounter another transformative concept: "Being Coachable." While closely related to the willingness to learn, being coachable encompasses distinct qualities that set it apart as a crucial element for achieving excellence in various aspects of life.

To grasp the true essence of being coachable, let's explore the key differences between "Being Willing to Learn" and "Being Coachable."

Receiving Feedback with Openness

"Being Willing to Learn" emphasizes the importance of being receptive to new knowledge and insights. It involves seeking information actively and demonstrating curiosity. On the other hand, "Being Coachable" takes it a step further by embracing feedback with openness and humility. A coachable individual welcomes constructive criticism, acknowledging that it is a powerful tool for self-improvement. When you're open to feedback, your brain is open and doesn't immediately close.

I, myself, have thought or even said out loud, "That will never work," before even contemplating the idea. Don't close your mind so quickly.

Active Application of Guidance

While "Being Willing to Learn" lays the groundwork for acquiring knowledge, "Being Coachable" involves actively applying that knowledge to refine skills and behaviors. Coachable individuals actively seek guidance and mentorship, understanding that mere accumulation of knowledge is not enough; its application is the catalyst for growth.

Seeking Mentors and Coaches

Being willing to learn can lead to self-directed learning through books, courses, or online resources. In contrast, being coachable involves actively seeking mentors and coaches who can provide personalized guidance. A coachable person recognizes the value of learning from others' experiences and benefits from the wisdom imparted by those who have walked similar paths.

There are people in your field, area of study/interest, or profession who are willing to help. You just need to ask.

Embracing Vulnerability

"Being Willing to Learn" might involve a degree of vulnerability in acknowledging areas for improvement. However, "Being Coachable" takes vulnerability to a deeper level. It means exposing oneself to critique and being receptive to change, even when it challenges long-held beliefs or habits. When you think you know it all, that is when you have to stop, listen, and learn.

Initiating Self-Reflection

Being coachable extends beyond external guidance; it also involves an ongoing process of self-reflection. Coachable individuals proactively assess their actions, choices, and behaviors, seeking opportunities for growth and development.

Implementing and Adapting

While both concepts value learning, "Being Willing to Learn" might stop at the acquisition of knowledge. In contrast, "Being Coachable" emphasizes implementing what is learned and adapting as necessary. This action-oriented approach results in tangible progress and continuous improvement.

Eagerness for Growth

A willingness to learn is a mindset, whereas being coachable reflects an eagerness for growth and the determination to reach one's full potential. Coachable individuals display a hunger for improvement, constantly striving to better themselves.

In summary, "Being Willing to Learn" is the foundation upon which "Being Coachable" is built. The former involves openness to new knowledge and experiences, while the latter takes it a step further by embracing feedback, seeking mentors, and actively applying what is learned. Being coachable requires a combination of humility, vulnerability, and a proactive approach to self-improvement.

In your journey to a "Happy New You!" remember that both being willing to learn and being coachable are invaluable traits necessary for growth. Embrace the power of learning, seek guidance, and apply the insights gained. By being coachable, you open the door to transformative growth and set yourself on a path toward greatness.

In the following chapters, we will explore practical strategies for cultivating coachability and unlocking your potential for unparalleled success. Get ready to embrace the power of being coachable as we continue on this transformative journey towards becoming the best version of yourself.

> "THE BREATH IS THE ULTIMATE KEY TO YOUR WELL-BEING, AND IF DONE RIGHT, IT HAS THE POWER TO TRANSFORM YOUR ENTIRE LIFE PHYSICAL, MENTAL, AND SPIRITUAL.
>
> — TONY ROBBINS

CHAPTER 3

BREATHE - HARNESSING THE POWER OF DEEP DIAPHRAGMATIC BREATHING

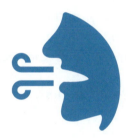

In the midst of our fast-paced lives, a profound tool for relaxation and calmness resides within us - the power of deep diaphragmatic breathing. Something so simple yet forgotten. In this chapter, we'll explore the transformative practice that can bring harmony to your mind, body, and soul.

The Art of Deep Diaphragmatic Breathing

Deep diaphragmatic breathing involves using the diaphragm to draw breath deep into the lungs, filling them to their fullest capacity. This intentional practice engages the parasympathetic nervous system, triggering a relaxation response that counters the stress-induced activation of the sympathetic nervous system.

The Lymphatic System and Deep Breathing

One of the many benefits of deep diaphragmatic breathing lies in its positive impact on the lymphatic system. Often referred to as the body's sewerage system, the lymphatic system plays a vital role in protecting each cell by removing dead cells, blood proteins, and toxins from the body. Deep breaths assist the lymphatic system in clearing out these waste materials.

Benefits Of Deep Breathing

Deep abdominal breathing causes full oxygen exchange, bringing in oxygen and taking out carbon dioxide. This, in turn, will slow the heartbeat and lower blood pressure. Deep breathing activates the parasympathetic (calming) nervous system, taking you out of fight/flight, reducing anxiety, and improving digestion. Increased cognition, concentration, and focus will be achieved after practicing deep breathing on a regular basis.

> "When you own your breath, nobody can steal your peace."
>
> **Unknown**

The Deep Breathing Technique - A Practice for Vitality

Follow these steps to engage in the powerful deep breathing technique:

1. Find a comfortable, quiet place to sit or lie down. Place one hand on your chest and the other on your abdomen.
2. Inhale deeply through your nose, allowing your abdomen and lower rib cage to expand. Feel the breath filling your lungs as your chest rises slightly.
3. Exhale slowly through your mouth, focusing on completely emptying your lungs. Feel your abdomen and chest falling as you release your breath.

4. Continue this deep breathing pattern, inhaling for a count of 4, holding for a count of 16, and exhaling for a count of 8.
5. Practice this technique for 5 to 10 minutes daily, ideally in the morning, evening, and before bed.

Embrace the power of deep diaphragmatic breathing as a foundational practice for relaxation, rejuvenation, and enhanced well-being. With each conscious breath, you can unlock the potential for inner peace and vitality. As you inhale, envision yourself drawing in positivity and calmness. As you exhale, let go of stress and tension, inviting a sense of balance into your life.

> "PURE WATER IS THE WORLD'S FIRST AND FOREMOST MEDICINE.
>
> SLOVAKIAN PROVERB"

CHAPTER 4

HYDRATION - QUENCHING YOUR BODY'S THIRST FOR VITALITY

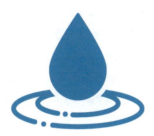

In the hustle and bustle of our daily lives, we often overlook one of the simplest yet most essential elements of human existence - water. In this chapter, we will explore the profound importance of water and the alarming reality that many of us may be going through each day more dehydrated than we realize.

Your Body's Cry for Hydration

Dr. Fereydoon Batmanghelidj, a renowned physician, emphasized in his book "Your Body's Many Cries for Water" - the critical role water plays in maintaining our health and well-being. Our bodies are comprised of approximately 60% water, and this life-sustaining substance is involved in almost every bodily function, from regulating temperature to aiding digestion and transporting nutrients.

Unveiling the Symptoms of Dehydration

Dehydration occurs when the body loses more water than it takes in, and this imbalance can lead to a range of health issues. Surprisingly, many common ailments, such as headaches, fatigue, vertigo, and difficulty concentrating, may be linked to mild dehydration. Recognizing the signs of dehydration can help us address this fundamental aspect of our health.

Urine Color and Frequency: By the time you feel thirsty, your body might already be in the early stages of dehydration. Relying solely on thirst as a cue to drink water might not be sufficient to maintain optimal hydration. Some people who are dehydrated don't even feel thirsty. Urine color can give insight into dehydration. If your urine is dark, then you are headed towards dehydration. For most people, urinating 6-7 times per day is normal. If you are doing less than that, you could become dehydrated.

Low Energy and Fatigue: Dehydration can lead to reduced energy levels and feelings of tiredness. Low blood volume from dehydration causes your heart to pump harder, expending extra energy, which in turn will make you more fatigued. Staying hydrated can help you feel more energized throughout the day.

Difficulty Concentrating: Inadequate water intake can impair cognitive function and focus. It can make you feel spaced out or give you brain fog. If you are significantly dehydrated, you could feel dizzy when you move your head. Even mild dehydration of 2% can affect memory, concentration, and reaction time. Keeping your brain hydrated can enhance mental clarity and performance.

Headaches and Migraines: Dehydration is a common trigger for headaches and migraines. When you are dehydrated, your brain shrinks, pulling away from the skull and triggering the pain receptors in the lining of the brain called the meninges. Proper hydration may help reduce the frequency and intensity of these painful episodes.

Dry Skin and Bad Breath: Lack of water can result in dry skin and contribute to bad breath. Dehydration can cause your skin to feel tight and look dull. A quick and easy test for skin dehydration is the pinch test. Pinch your skin over the back of your hand, and if it is slow to return to its normal state, you might be dehydrated. Or you can do the nailbed press test. Push on a nail until it turns white, then let go. It should take 2 seconds or less to turn pink again. If it takes over 2 seconds, then you also might be dehydrated. Proper hydration can promote healthy skin and oral hygiene.

The Power of Staying Hydrated

Maintaining proper hydration is essential for overall well-being and vitality. Consider these benefits of staying hydrated:

Optimal Physical Performance: Proper hydration supports physical performance by improving endurance, strength, and coordination. It helps regulate temperature so that you don't overheat while exercising.

Healthy Digestion: Water aids in the digestion process, helping your body absorb essential nutrients and remove waste.

Joint Health: Adequate hydration supports joint lubrication and reduces the risk of joint-related discomfort. The cartilage in the joints is 60-80% water, and being hydrated helps bring in needed nutrients.

Detoxification: Water is essential for flushing out toxins and waste products from the body, promoting better overall detoxification.

Regulated Body Temperature: Staying hydrated helps regulate body temperature, preventing overheating during physical activity or hot weather.

The Hydration Habit

To ensure that you are adequately hydrated, establish a habit of drinking water throughout the day. Carry a reusable water bottle with you and take sips regularly, even if you don't feel thirsty. Remember that individual hydration needs may vary, and factors like climate, activity level, and age can influence your water intake requirements. A simple formula is to drink ½ your body weight in ounces. If you weigh 100 pounds, then you will drink 50 ounces. I typically get 80-90 ounces per day and feel good at that level, but when I am in a dry area with low humidity, I drink 120-130 ounces per day.

Embrace the power of water as a foundational pillar of health. By quenching your body's thirst and staying properly hydrated, you unleash a wellspring of vitality that fuels your journey toward a "Happy New You!" Let the flow of hydration be a constant reminder of the life-sustaining force within you, supporting your well-being in mind, body, and spirit.

> **SLEEP IS THAT GOLDEN CHAIN THAT TIES HEALTH AND OUR BODIES TOGETHER.**
>
> THOMAS DEKKER

CHAPTER 5
EMBRACING THE POWER OF RESTFUL SLEEP

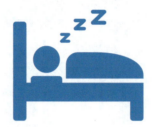

In the quest for a "Happy New You!" and a life of vitality, one fundamental aspect often gets neglected in our fast-paced world - the gift of restful sleep. In this chapter, we will delve into the transformative power of sleep and uncover its profound impact on our physical, mental, and emotional well-being.

Sleep - The Foundation of Vitality

Sleep is not merely a time of rest but a foundational pillar of health that allows our bodies and minds to rejuvenate, heal, and thrive. While we may prioritize exercise, nutrition, and other aspects of wellness, it's essential to recognize that quality sleep is equally vital for optimal functioning. In fact, if you do everything right but don't get enough sleep you will not have the good health you are working towards.

The Science of Sleep

Sleep is a complex physiological process that involves several stages, each serving a unique purpose. Rapid Eye Movement (REM) and Non-Rapid Eye Movement (NREM) sleep cycles work together to promote brain health, memory consolidation, and emotional regulation.

During NREM sleep, the body repairs tissues releases growth hormones, and boosts the immune system. REM sleep, on the other hand, plays a crucial role in processing emotions, solidifying memories, and enhancing creativity. Since we do most of our healing while we sleep, it is critical to get at least 7 hours of sleep per night.

The Alarming Impact of Sleep Deprivation

Unfortunately, the modern lifestyle often leads to insufficient sleep, and the consequences can be far-reaching. Chronic sleep deprivation not only impairs cognitive function and emotional well-being but also increases the risk of various health issues, including obesity, cardiovascular disease, and compromised immune function. It is also known that more people get into automobile collisions due to sleep deprivation.

The Sleep-Health Connection

Quality sleep has a profound impact on both physical and mental health:

Enhanced Cognitive Function: Restful sleep improves concentration, attention, and problem-solving abilities, fostering enhanced cognitive performance.

Emotional Resilience: Sufficient sleep supports emotional resilience, helping us navigate stress and challenges with greater ease. We all know the world is a harder place to be in when we haven't had sleep.

Improved Immune Function: During sleep, the immune system fights infections and promotes healing, strengthening our defenses against illnesses. Sleep is the number one way I keep from getting sick. When everyone around me is getting sick I make sure I get to sleep on time.

Physical Recovery and Repair: Sleep is a time for the body to repair tissues, rebuild muscles, and recharge energy stores. When you sleep deep, your blood flow increases and growth hormones are released, repairing and growing muscles.

Mental and Emotional Balance: Adequate sleep supports emotional regulation and reduces the risk of mood disorders. Getting into REM sleep helps the brain process emotional information, especially consolidating positive emotional content.

> "Sleep is an investment in the energy you need to be effective tomorrow."
>
> **Tom Roth.**

Cultivating Healthy Sleep Habits

To embrace the power of restful sleep, consider incorporating these habits into your nightly routine:

Consistent Sleep Schedule: Aim for a regular sleep schedule, going to bed and waking up at the same time each day, even on weekends.

Create a Soothing Sleep Environment: Make your bedroom a sleep sanctuary - comfortable, cool, and free from distractions. Try to get your bedroom as dark as possible. Get blackout curtains and put electrical tape over lights such as alarm systems, alarm clocks, and smoke detectors. Keep your room temperature between 60-68 degrees, as a room that is too cold or warm doesn't allow for good restful sleep.

Limit Screen Time Before Bed: Minimize exposure to screens and bright lights before bedtime to promote the release of the sleep-inducing hormone melatonin. If you must be on your phone/computer, you can get blue-blocking sunglasses or set your phone to night mode.

Relaxation Techniques: Practice relaxation techniques like deep breathing, meditation, or gentle stretching to unwind before sleep. Counting sheep or counting from 100 can help you unwind and fall asleep.

Mindful Nutrition: Avoid heavy meals, caffeine, and stimulants before bedtime. Caffeine should be stopped by noon, and your last meal of the day should be at least 2 hours prior to going to sleep. You can drink tea with calming herbs such as Ashwagandha, Tulsi (Holy Basil), passionflower, or chamomile to help calm you down and get ready for sleep. I take magnesium before bed, which helps with brain and muscle relaxation.

Embrace the power of restful sleep as a cornerstone of vitality. By honoring your body's need for rejuvenating rest, you unlock the full potential for a "Happy New You!" Each night becomes an opportunity to embrace healing, transformation, and renewal as you awaken to a life of boundless energy and well-being.

> **YOU CANNOT HAVE A POSITIVE LIFE AND A NEGATIVE MIND**
>
> — JOYCE MEYER

CHAPTER 6

MINDFUL CONSUMPTION - GI/GO

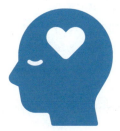

In our journey towards a "Happy New You!" and a life of vitality, we must recognize the profound connection between restful sleep and mindful consumption. As sleep nourishes our body and mind, so does the content we choose to fill our minds with daily. In this chapter, we will explore the significance of being aware of what we consume mentally and its transformative impact on our overall well-being.

Garbage in, Garbage Out - The Power of Mindful Consumption

The phrase "Garbage in, Garbage Out" (GI/GO) is a powerful concept that originated in the world of computer science. It highlights the idea that the quality of input determines the quality of output. In computing, if you input faulty or irrelevant data, the output will be flawed or inaccurate. Similarly, in the realm of our mental well-being, what we feed our minds greatly influences our thoughts, emotions, and overall outlook on life.

The Impact of Negative Content

Endless exposure to negative news, fear-inducing stories, and doom and gloom can take a toll on our mental, physical, and emotional health. Consuming this type of content can lead to increased stress, anxiety, and a pessimistic outlook on life, in addition to headaches, neck pain and back pain. The constant barrage of distressing information can leave us feeling overwhelmed and emotionally drained. Recognizing the significance of the content we expose ourselves to and its potential consequences on our well-being is essential. If you find yourself being grumpy, angry, or frustrated, check what information you are reading or watching. My bet is that it isn't anything positive.

The Power of Positive Input

On the other hand, filling our minds with positive and uplifting content can have a transformative effect. Consuming inspirational stories, educational materials, and content that promotes growth and well-being can elevate our mood, boost our resilience, and inspire us to lead fulfilling lives. Positive input nourishes our minds and cultivates a sense of hope and optimism, even in challenging times.

Mindful Consumption for a Healthy Mind

Limit Exposure to Negative News: Be mindful of your time watching or reading negative news. While staying informed is important, consider setting boundaries to avoid immersing yourself in a constant stream of distressing content. Choose specific times to catch up on news updates and balance it with other positive activities. Personally, I can only look at headlines 1-2 times per week as negative news is so distressing to me that I find myself becoming depressed, anxious, and less hopeful.

Choose Uplifting Content: Seek out positive and inspiring content that adds value to your life. Follow educational channels, read uplifting books, and surround yourself with positive influences. Watch funny and uplifting TV shows or movies. Fill your social media feed with accounts that share motivational messages, personal growth tips, and content that sparks joy. When I have had a tough day, I look at cute dog and cat videos. I am feeling my stress release by watching several minutes of these sweet animals.

Mind Your Social Media Feed: Curate your social media feed to include content that supports your growth and well-being. Unfollow accounts that bring negativity into your life. Engage with online communities focusing on positivity, personal development, and empowerment.

Practice Mindfulness: Develop a habit of mindful consumption. Before watching or reading something, pause and consider how it might impact your mood and well-being. If you notice negative emotions arising, redirect your focus to more positive content or engaging activities.

Nourish Your Mind Before Sleep: Before bedtime, opt for calming and positive content that can help you unwind and promote restful sleep. Read a good book, listen to calming music. Avoid engaging with stressful or intense material close to bedtime, as it may, and most likely will, affect the quality of your sleep.

The Power of Choice

Remember that you have the power to choose what you fill your mind with. Take ownership of your mental well-being by consciously selecting content that aligns with your values, aspirations, and overall sense of well-being. Surround yourself with sources that inspire you, uplift your spirit, and foster personal growth.

I hear people all day long who say they are stressed out but won't stop watching the news. They say they have to stay informed. What is more important to you- good sleep, a calm brain or anxiety and being informed? You have the power to choose.

Embrace the power of mindful consumption as you embrace restful sleep. By being aware of what you fill your mind with, you can create a nurturing environment that supports your growth, positivity, and well-being. As you choose to focus on uplifting content, you nurture a "Happy New You!" and a life of mental clarity, emotional resilience, and inspiration. By consciously selecting the content you consume, you become the steward of your mental landscape, cultivating a mindset that empowers you to face life's challenges with courage and optimism. Let this intentional approach to mindful consumption guide your path to a more fulfilling and enriched existence.

> **TO EAT IS A NECESSITY, BUT TO EAT INTELLIGENTLY IS AN ART.**
>
> — FRANÇOIS DE LA ROCHEFOUCAULD

CHAPTER 7
THE POWER OF ALKALIZING FOODS - NOURISHING YOUR BODY'S BALANCE

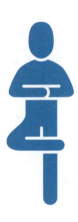

In our journey towards a "Happy New You!" and a life of vitality, the foods we consume are crucial in determining our overall well-being. Among the various dietary approaches, the concept of alkalizing foods has gained attention for its potential health benefits. However, it's important to clarify that embracing alkalizing foods doesn't mean adopting a strict vegetarian or vegan lifestyle. Rather, it's about incorporating more alkaline-rich foods into our diet to nourish our body's balance and promote optimal health.

Understanding Alkalizing Foods

Alkalizing foods are those that have an alkaline effect on the body, meaning they can help balance our internal pH level. This balance is crucial because the modern Western diet tends to be high in acidic foods, which can potentially disrupt our body's natural equilibrium. On the other hand, alkalizing foods are typically rich in essential vitamins, minerals, and antioxidants that contribute to our well-being.

The Benefits of Alkalizing Foods

Incorporating alkalizing foods into our diet can offer several potential benefits:

Enhanced Digestion: Alkaline-rich foods, such as leafy greens, avocados, and cucumbers, are often easier for our digestive system to process, promoting better nutrient absorption and gut health.

Reduced Inflammation: A diet with a higher pH balance may help reduce chronic inflammation linked to various health conditions. Foods like almonds, broccoli, and kale are excellent choices in this regard. I often feel puffiness in people's tissues, and then it will reduce. I ask them what has changed, and they usually tell me they changed their diet and added more vegetables.

Support for Bone Health: Some health advocates suggest that an alkaline diet might support bone health and reduce the risk of osteoporosis. Nourishing your body with alkalizing foods like pears, raspberries, and sesame seeds can contribute to bone health. I wasn't able to find any research studies about alkaline foods helping bone loss, but it is interesting that a study shows alkaline water may help with bone loss.

Boosted Energy Levels: Alkalizing foods provide a steady energy source, contributing to sustained vitality throughout the day.

Foods like quinoa, sweet potatoes, and chia seeds are energizing and delicious additions to your meals.

Practical Tips for Embracing Alkalizing Foods

It's essential to remember that incorporating alkalizing foods into our diet is not an all-or-nothing approach. Here are some practical tips to help you embrace the power of alkaline-rich foods.

Add More Fruits and Vegetables: Make an effort to include a variety of fruits and vegetables in your meals. These plant-based foods are naturally alkaline and rich in essential nutrients. Try spinach and strawberry salad, roasted Brussels sprouts, or a colorful fruit and leafy green smoothie. I would like to state that fruits are eaten way more than vegetables. They are always lumped together, so I have started asking people if they eat their vegetables. You can get too much of nature's candy: fruit.

Meatless Mondays: Consider practicing "Meatless Mondays" or other similar approaches. These designated days allow your body to enjoy a mini-vacation from meat and explore the diverse world of plant-based meals. Prepare a flavorful vegetable stir-fry, hearty lentil soup, or a mouthwatering mushroom risotto. When I say plant-based meals, I mean meals designed with vegetables, fruits, nuts, and seeds, not factory-made fake meat "foods."

Hydration with Alkaline Water: Explore drinking alkaline water with a slightly higher pH level than regular water. Staying hydrated with alkaline water can complement your efforts to nourish your body's balance. Add slices of lemon or cucumber to your water for a refreshing twist.

Balance is Key: While incorporating alkalizing foods is beneficial, it's essential to maintain a balanced diet that includes a variety of foods from different food groups. Pair your alkaline-rich meals with a source of protein, such as grilled chicken, fish, or tofu, to create well-rounded and satisfying dishes.

Embrace the power of alkalizing foods to nourish your body's balance and promote overall wellness. By gradually incorporating more fruits, vegetables, and other alkaline-rich foods into your diet, you support your body's natural equilibrium and lay the groundwork for a "Happy New You!" Let this be a journey of exploration and self-discovery as you discover the flavors and benefits of alkalizing foods, enhancing your well-being one nourishing and yummy bite at a time.

> "PHYSICAL FITNESS IS NOT ONLY ONE OF THE MOST IMPORTANT KEYS TO A HEALTH BODY, IT IS THE BASIS OF DYNAMIC AND CREATIVE INTELLECTUAL ACTIVITY.
>
> — JOHN F. KENNEDY"

CHAPTER 8

EMBRACE THE POWER OF DAILY MOVEMENT

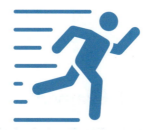

The importance of staying active cannot be overstated in our pursuit of a "Happy New You!" and a life of vitality. The phrase "Move It Or Lose It" holds profound wisdom, reminding us that consistent movement is essential for physical and mental well-being. You don't need to be an advanced yogi or a master of Qi Gong to reap the benefits of daily activity. In this chapter, we will explore how incorporating just 5 to 10 minutes of simple movements into your daily routine can significantly affect your overall health and happiness.

The Power of Daily Activity

Regular physical activity is not only vital for maintaining a healthy weight but also has numerous other benefits:

Enhanced Flexibility: Simple movements can improve flexibility, making it easier to perform daily tasks and reducing the risk of injuries.

Boosted Mood: Exercise stimulates the release of endorphins, our body's natural mood elevators, promoting feelings of joy and reducing stress and anxiety.

Improved Circulation: Physical activity gets your blood flowing, nourishing your body with oxygen and nutrients while aiding in the removal of waste products.

Heart Health: Regular movement supports cardiovascular health, lowering the risk of heart disease and improving overall cardiovascular fitness.

Embracing Simple Movements

You don't need a gym membership or fancy equipment to get moving. Incorporating simple movements into your daily routine is easy and can be done in the comfort of your home. Here are some ideas to help you get started:

Morning Stretches: Begin your day with gentle stretches, reaching for the sky, touching your toes, and moving your body to wake up your muscles. Most mornings, I do stretches even before getting out of bed. I bring my knees to my chest, let one leg drop off the side of the bed, and reach up and out with my arms and legs.

Short Walks: Take a 5-minute walk outside during your lunch break or after dinner. Fresh air and a change of scenery can do wonders for your mood. Short walks are a great way to clear your head during your workday. You might even come up with a million-dollar idea.

Dance Breaks: Turn on your favorite music and have a dance party in your living room. Let loose and let the music move you. This one is so easy, as many of you work from home. No one can see you dance your heart out.

Chair Exercises: If you spend most of your day sitting, incorporate chair exercises into your routine. Try seated leg lifts, shoulder rolls, and arm circles.

Yoga or Qi Gong: If you're interested in trying more structured movements, consider beginner-friendly yoga or Qi Gong videos available online. Many videos vary from 5 to 15 minutes, which would be perfect for a work break.

Easy Movements: Some easy ways to get movement in your day while at work are to have a headset on during a meeting, walk around your office, and get up whenever you print something on the copier. Parking farther away from the door either to work or when you go to the grocery store helps with getting daily movement.

> "Exercise is a celebration of what your body can do, not a punishment for what you ate."
>
> **Unknown.**

The Power of Consistency

The key to reaping the benefits of daily activity lies in consistency. Aim to incorporate 5 to 10 minutes of movement into your daily schedule, making it a non-negotiable part of your routine. By committing to this practice, you'll experience a positive transformation in your physical and mental well-being.

Start Your Movement Ritual

Think of these daily movement moments as a way to honor your body and show it some love. Create a "movement ritual" that suits your schedule and preferences. It could be as simple as stretching when you wake up, taking a walk during your lunch break, and having a dance break before dinner. By making movement a regular part of your day, you'll notice a positive shift in your energy levels, mood, and overall well-being.

Embrace the power of daily activity and honor your body by moving it regularly. Remember, you don't have to be an expert or spend hours at the gym to make a difference. Dedicating just a few minutes each day to simple movements will nurture a "Happy New You!" and build the foundation for a life filled with vitality and well-being. Let the joy of movement become a daily ritual, enhancing your physical health and uplifting your spirit, one step or stretch at a time.

> **A HEALTHY OUTSIDE STARTS FROM THE INSIDE.**
>
> ROBERT URICH

CHAPTER 9
GET THINGS MOVING - NURTURING REGULAR BOWEL HEALTH

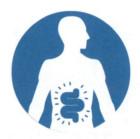

In our pursuit of optimal health and a "Happy New You!" one essential aspect that is often overlooked is the regularity of our bowel movements. The state of our digestive system profoundly influences our overall well-being, yet many shy away from discussing it openly. It's time to shed light on this vital topic and explore natural and healthy ways to support regular bowel movements.

Understanding Bowel Health

A well-functioning digestive system is crucial for the proper absorption of nutrients and the elimination of waste products. Regular bowel movements are a sign of a healthy digestive tract. However, many factors can disrupt bowel regularity, including dietary choices, stress, sedentary lifestyles, and inadequate hydration.

Embracing Natural Approaches

When it comes to supporting regular bowel movements, there are natural and healthy steps we can take. Let's explore some of them:

Dietary Fiber: Including fiber-rich foods in your diet can promote bowel regularity. We need foods that have soluble and insoluble fiber for our digestion. Both are helpful with constipation. Soluble fiber dissolves in water, feeds our good gut bacteria, improves blood sugar and cholesterol, and regulates bowel function. Some foods with soluble fiber are oats, oat bran, barley, nuts, seeds, beans, lentils, peas, apples, oranges, and psyllium. Insoluble fiber adds bulk to the stool and helps the food pass through the digestive tract more quickly. Some of the insoluble fiber foods are nuts, cauliflower, green beans, blackberries, potatoes, celery, parsnips, cucumbers, and whole grains.

Stay Hydrated: Drinking adequate water daily helps keep stool soft and easy to pass. Aim for at least eight glasses of water daily or ½ your body weight in ounces.

Regular Exercise: Physical activity stimulates bowel movements by encouraging the natural contraction and relaxation of the intestinal muscles. Engaging in regular exercises such as:

Walking: A brisk walk for 15-30 minutes daily can help get things moving.

Yoga: Gentle yoga poses, such as seated twists, bow poses, and forward bends, can aid digestion and bowel movements.

Abdominal Exercises: Movements that engage the core, like leg lifts, crunches, dead bugs, and bicycle crunches, can stimulate the digestive system. Most days, I do belly contractions for several minutes before I go to sleep. I contract my belly like I am trying to get my belly button away from my waistband, then I hold it for 5-10 seconds, and I repeat it several times.

I learned a great abdominal exercise from an amazing physical therapist, Jeff Powney, PT. I will use this one also for abdominal contraction and abdominal massage. You start on the floor on all fours. If you can't get on the floor, you can hold onto a counter and mimic being on the floor. You take a big breath in, your belly expands, then let the breath out and follow it all the way out with your belly- your belly should be moving away from your waistband. Take another deep breath in and out, and try to make your belly smaller. Your contraction should be stronger than the last one. Please take a deep breath, let it out, and follow it with your belly again. Your belly should be working towards being sucked in. Hold the contraction and roll your belly like a belly dancer for 10 seconds, then relax. Your belly has now massaged your colon.

The Squatty Potty: For those seeking an additional way to promote regular bowel movements, the Squatty Potty may be worth considering. The Squatty Potty is a simple stool that fits around the base of your toilet, allowing you to elevate your feet slightly while using the bathroom. This posture mimics a more natural squatting position, relaxing the colon and making elimination easier. Many people find the Squatty Potty to be a helpful aid in maintaining bowel regularity.

The Path to Bowel Wellness

We can embark on a path to bowel wellness by embracing natural and healthy practices. Regular bowel movements reflect our inner health, and by paying attention to this often-neglected aspect of our well-being, we can achieve a more vibrant and energetic life.

Incorporate fiber-rich foods and hydrate yourself adequately to support digestive health. Engage in regular physical activity, whether a brisk walk, gentle yoga, or abdominal exercises, to stimulate the digestive system. And for those looking to try something new, consider the Squatty Potty as a potential aid.

Together, these steps can pave the way to regular bowel health, supporting your journey to a "Happy New You!" with vitality and well-being. Remember, your health is a precious gift, and taking care of your digestive system is an empowering step towards a healthier and more fulfilling life.

> **YOU TAKE THE HEALTHIEST DIET IN THE WORLD. IF YOU GAVE THOSE PEOPLE VITAMINS, THEY WOULD BE TWICE AS HEALTHY. SO VITAMINS ARE VALUABLE.**
>
> ―ROBERT ATKINS

CHAPTER 10
THE ESSENTIAL VITAMINS YOU NEED

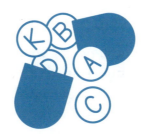

In our quest for optimal health and a "Happy New You!" incorporating essential vitamins into our daily routine is a powerful step towards nourishing our bodies. While the world of supplements can be overwhelming, we want to focus on a straightforward approach that yields substantial benefits without overwhelming you with excessive pills.

Let's explore the top three essential supplements that can significantly affect the average person's well-being.

A High-Quality Multi-Vitamin

A high-quality multivitamin can be a safety net, ensuring you receive a broad spectrum of essential vitamins and minerals. Even if you strive to maintain a balanced diet, there may be gaps in your nutrient intake, and studies show that our soil is getting depleted, so our food doesn't have the nutrition levels that it used to have.

A multivitamin helps fill those gaps and supports various bodily functions, from energy production to immune system health.

Vitamin D - The Sunshine Vitamin

Vitamin D is a superstar nutrient, often called the "sunshine vitamin", because our bodies can produce it when exposed to sunlight. However, many spend less time outdoors due to modern lifestyles, leading to widespread vitamin D deficiencies. Vitamin D receptors are found in nearly all, if not all, cells in the body, making it a crucial nutrient to be sufficient in. It is necessary for many bodily functions that we don't even realize, such as hair loss.

Unfortunately, most insurance companies do not want to pay for lab tests for vitamin D, but it needs to be done. I have known people who were so low <10 when you should be up towards 60. With a number that low, a person is not thriving.

Vitamin D plays a crucial role in:

- Bone And Muscular Health: Vitamin D is necessary for calcium absorption, maintaining strong bones and reducing your chance of bone fractures and osteoporosis. Reduced calcium absorption due to Vitamin D deficiency also is a cause of muscle pain and weakness.
- Immune Function: Vitamin D helps modulate immune responses, supporting your body's defense against infections and illnesses. A study published in the Journal of the American Medical Association found that Vitamin D supplementation may significantly reduce the risk of respiratory infections.
- Mood and Well-Being: Emerging research suggests adequate vitamin D levels may positively influence mood and mental health. Low vitamin D has been linked to fatigue, depression, and low mood. This is most likely why the northern states have a high percentage of people

taking antidepressants. I would go to Vegas in the dark months for years and just soak up the sun. I could feel my mood changing.

Omega-3 Fatty Acids

Omega-3 fatty acids are essential fats our bodies need but cannot produce independently. They are crucial for heart health, brain function, and inflammation regulation. While you can obtain omega-3s from certain foods like fatty fish (salmon, mackerel, sardines), walnuts, and flaxseeds, a high-quality fish oil supplement can be a convenient way to ensure an adequate intake of these beneficial fats. With fish oil supplements, getting a good quality supplement is vital. It isn't good if it tastes fishy and causes you to burp fish.

Quality Matters

When choosing supplements, quality matters. Look for products from reputable brands that undergo rigorous testing for purity, potency, and absence of contaminants. Cheaper is not the way to go with fish oils. Taking a cheap, most likely rancid fish oil is worse than not taking them at all.

The Balanced Approach

While these three supplements can form a solid foundation for your health regimen, remember that they do not replace a healthy diet and lifestyle. Nourishing your body with whole, nutrient-dense foods, staying hydrated, and engaging in regular physical activity are all essential components of a vibrant and well-balanced life.

Empower Your Health with Essential Vitamins

Taking the right supplements can empower your health and well-being, giving you the support you need to thrive in your daily life. Embrace the simplicity of a high-quality multivitamin, boost your vitamin D levels with a sunshine supplement, and include omega-3 fatty acids to support your heart and brain health. As you take these steps, remember that the path to optimal health is balanced, nourishing your body and mind with a holistic approach.

> **THE MORE THAT YOU READ, THE MORE THINGS YOU WILL KNOW. THE MORE THAT YOU LEARN, THE MORE PLACES YOU'LL GO.**
>
> ― DR. SEUSS

CHAPTER 11
UNLEASH THE POWER OF READING - IGNITE YOUR PATH TO SUCCESS

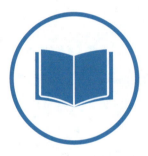

In the journey of becoming a "Happy New You!" and achieving personal growth, few practices rival the transformative power of reading. Embracing the wisdom of renowned figures like Jim Rohn and Brian Tracy, this chapter will illuminate the importance of reading and how it can unlock doors to success, knowledge, and self-discovery.

"Miss a Meal, But Don't Miss a Book" - Jim Rohn

Jim Rohn's timeless quote captures the essence of the impact that reading can have on our lives. "Miss a meal if you have to, but don't miss a book." These words remind us that the nourishment gained from reading goes beyond physical sustenance; it feeds our minds and souls, igniting the flame of knowledge and inspiration within us.

Readers Are Leaders

The phrase "Readers are leaders" underscores the profound connection between reading and leadership. Reading allows us to learn from the experiences and insights of others, inspiring us to lead with wisdom and empathy. Through books, we can access humanity's collective wisdom, honing our decision-making abilities and guiding us on the path to leadership excellence.

The Brian Tracy Perspective

Brian Tracy, a renowned author and motivational speaker, echoes the significance of consistent reading in his quote: "If you read one hour per day in your field, that will translate into about one book per week. One book per week translates into about 50 books per year. Over the next ten years, 50 books per year will translate into about 500 books."

You can exponentially expand your knowledge and expertise by dedicating just one hour a day to reading in your chosen field. The accumulation of wisdom from 500 books over a decade empowers you to approach challenges with a heightened level of insight and a depth of understanding that sets you apart as a true leader in your field.

The Power of Lifelong Learning

Reading is a portal to the boundless realm of lifelong learning. It allows us to delve into diverse subjects, explore new perspectives, and constantly evolve as individuals. As we embrace reading, we open ourselves to personal growth and self-discovery, tapping into the vast reservoir of human knowledge and experience.

Reading Fuels Imagination

Beyond gaining knowledge, reading sparks our imagination and creativity. Books transport us to different worlds, eras, and realities, expanding the horizons of our minds. Through literature, we can empathize with characters, envision new possibilities, and embrace the magic of storytelling.

Practical Tips to Cultivate a Reading Habit

Set Reading Goals: Determine how much time you can dedicate to reading each day or week and set achievable reading goals. Aim to read a certain number of books in a year, reflecting on your progress regularly. My life is extremely busy, but I always make time for reading. I typically get 10-15 minutes of reading right before going to sleep.

Create a Reading Space: Designate a comfortable and inviting space for reading, free from distractions, where you can immerse yourself in the world of books.

Diversify Your Reading List: Explore various genres, from fiction to non-fiction, self-help, biographies, and more. Diversifying your reading list enhances your perspective and enriches your understanding of the world.

Discuss and Share: Engage in book discussions with friends, family, or clubs. Sharing your thoughts and insights can deepen your understanding and appreciation of what you read.

Incorporating reading into your daily life is a transformative habit that will propel you toward growth and success. It enables you to lead with wisdom, cultivate creativity, and embrace lifelong learning. So, dive into the world of books, savor the knowledge they offer, and unlock the full potential of your mind as you journey toward becoming a leader in your own life and beyond. Remember, each page turned is a step closer to the best version of yourself, illuminating the path to a life of fulfilment and purpose.

> I WAKE UP IN THE MORNING, I DO A LITTLE STRETCHING EXERCISES, PICK UP THE HORN AND PLAY.
>
> — HERB ALPERT

CHAPTER 12

STRETCHING BEYOND LIMITS - EXPANDING BODY AND MIND

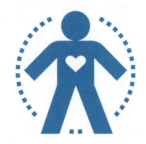

In our pursuit of a "Happy New You!" and a fulfilling life, we often find ourselves focusing on the physical aspects of health and well-being. However, we must not overlook the equally essential practice of stretching our minds and nurturing our mental agility. Just like we stretch our bodies to maintain flexibility, we can apply the same principle to our minds, leading to transformation and growth.

Stretching the Body - Embracing Flexibility

Stretching our bodies is key to maintaining physical flexibility and preventing injuries. It allows us to move freely, improves blood circulation, and helps relieve tension. Incorporating stretching exercises into our daily routine promotes overall health and enhances physical performance.

Examples of Body Stretching:

Yoga Practice: Engaging in yoga poses, such as downward dog, cobra, and warrior stretches, can improve flexibility, balance, and strength.

Dynamic Stretching: Before engaging in physical activities or workouts, perform dynamic stretches like leg swings, arm circles, and walking lunges to warm up your muscles and increase their range of motion.

Stretching the Mind - Expanding Horizons

Like the concept of stretching our bodies, stretching our minds is expanding our horizons, challenging our beliefs, and embracing new ideas. It's about breaking free from mental rigidity and embracing a growth mindset. The mind, like a rubber band, has the remarkable ability to stretch beyond its perceived limits.

> "The mind, once stretched by a new idea, never returns to its original dimensions."
>
> **Ralph Waldo Emerson**

Examples of Mind Expansion

Reading Diverse Books: Explore books from various genres, authors, and cultures to gain new perspectives and enrich your understanding of the world.

Learning a New Skill: Take up a new hobby, learn to play a musical instrument, or acquire a new language to stimulate your brain and expand your skill set.

The Growth Mindset

The growth mindset, popularized by psychologist Carol Dweck, emphasizes the belief that our abilities and intelligence can be developed through dedication and hard work. When we adopt a growth mindset, we view challenges as opportunities for learning and see failures as opportunities for success. This mindset empowers us to embrace change, welcome new perspectives, and continually evolve.

Stretching the Mind Through Learning

Continuous learning is one of the most effective ways to stretch our minds. Reading books, exploring diverse subjects, taking up new hobbies, taking classes in subjects that interest you, or engaging in thought-provoking discussions all contribute to expanding our mental faculties. Learning exposes us to new ideas, cultures, and ways of thinking, enriching our understanding of the world around us.

The Unstoppable Transformation

Just like a rubber band, or your underwear waistband, that never returns to its original shape once stretched pasts its limits, our minds are forever changed and expanded through the process of stretching. Embracing a mindset of continuous growth sets us on a path of unstoppable transformation, enabling us to face life's challenges with resilience and adaptability.

The Power of Mindful Stretching

Practicing mindful stretching involves being fully present in the moment and giving attention to our thoughts, feelings, and experiences. Mindful stretching encourages us to let go of limiting beliefs and cultivate self-awareness. It's a powerful practice that leads to greater clarity, focus, and emotional well-being.

Embrace the Stretch

As we incorporate stretching into our daily lives, both in our bodies and minds, we embrace the potential for extraordinary growth and change. Embrace the stretch, welcome the challenges, and expand your capabilities beyond what you ever thought possible.

In the journey of becoming a "Happy New You!" remember to stretch your body to stay flexible and active, and equally important, stretch your mind to embrace new perspectives and foster a growth mindset. By nurturing both physical and mental flexibility, you set yourself on a path of continuous self-improvement, embracing change, and expanding your horizons. Just like a rubber band, you'll discover that you can never return to your original shape, for you have forever been changed and transformed. Embrace the stretch, and let it empower you to reach new heights in every aspect of your life.

> **EVERY WALK WITH NATURE, ONE RECEIVES FAR MORE THAN HE SEEKS.**
>
> JOHN MUIR

CHAPTER 13

EMBRACE THE POWER OF WALKING - SMALL STEPS, BIG IMPACT

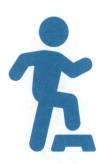

Walking is a simple yet transformative practice in the quest for a "Happy New You!" and a healthy lifestyle. We often hear about the "10,000 Steps Goal" as a benchmark for fitness, but the truth behind this number might surprise you. Originally popularized in Japan as a marketing ploy to sell pedometers, the 10,000 Steps Goal became a worldwide phenomenon. However, I want you to know that you don't have to be fixated on hitting this arbitrary number every single day; the goal is to just get out and walk.

The Power of Small Steps

The journey to an active and healthier life begins with small steps. The key is to start where you are and build upon daily repetitiveness. It's not about reaching some far-off finish line but the journey itself. Each step you take brings you closer to better health and well-being.

Tracking Your Progress

Documenting and tracking your progress can be a powerful motivator. It allows you to see how far you've come and gives you a sense of accomplishment. Whether you use a journal, a fitness app, or a simple spreadsheet, keeping track of your daily steps can help you stay on course and celebrate your achievements. A fun way to track your walking progress is to make a goal to walk to somewhere you always wanted to go, such as Spain. Have a map and plot the mileage as you go along and see how long it takes to get to your destination. You might never make it, but seeing how far you will get will be fun.

Walking Apps to Elevate Your Journey

Today, we have the advantage of technology that can take our walking goals to new heights. Numerous walking apps available for your smartphone can help you monitor and enhance your walking experience. Here are some popular ones to consider:

Step Tracker Apps: Apps like "Google Fit," "Apple Health," or "Fitbit" enable you to track your daily steps effortlessly. They offer intuitive interfaces, personalized goals, and progress insights.

Walking Route Apps: Discover new walking routes in your area with apps like "AllTrails" or "MapMyWalk." These apps provide maps, distances, and terrain details, making your walks more adventurous.

Community-Focused Apps: Join walking communities on apps like "Strava" or "Charity Miles" to connect with like-minded individuals and participate in virtual challenges for a sense of camaraderie and motivation.

Audio-Guided Walks: Enjoy audio-guided walking sessions with apps like "Aaptiv" or "Walking App - Walking for Weight Loss" that provide guidance, music, and inspiration as you stroll.

Small Daily Walking Goals

Here are some concrete examples of small daily walking goals that you can easily incorporate into your routine:

The Morning Stroll: Take a short walk around your neighborhood each morning to start your day on a positive note. Aim for 5-10 minutes to wake up your body and mind.

Lunch Break Wander: Instead of staying seated during your lunch break, take a 15-minute stroll around your workplace or nearby park. It will increase blood flow to your brain, boost your energy and refresh your focus for the afternoon.

Post-Dinner Walk: Enjoy a leisurely 10-15 minute walk with family or friends after dinner. It not only aids digestion but also provides an excellent opportunity for bonding and relaxation.

Park and Walk: When running errands, park a bit farther from the entrance to get some extra steps in. Embrace the chance to stretch your legs and take in the surroundings.

Walking Meetings: Opt for walking meetings with colleagues instead of sitting in a conference room if possible. The change of scenery can lead to more creativity and productivity.

Celebrate Your Progress

Remember, it's not about the number of steps you take each day; it's about making walking a regular part of your life. Celebrate your progress, no matter how small it may seem. Every step counts, and each day presents an opportunity to positively impact your health and well-being.

The Real Goal - Consistency

The real goal is consistency. By making walking a daily habit, you'll experience the cumulative benefits over time. Consistency is the key to building a strong foundation for a healthy and active lifestyle.

As you embrace the power of walking, let go of the pressure to reach a specific step count each day. Start small, build your routine, and track your progress along the way. Utilize walking apps to elevate your experience and make the journey more enjoyable.

Remember, it's about the journey, not the destination. Celebrate every step you take and keep moving forward, one stride at a time. The path to a "Happy New You!" is filled with small steps that lead to big changes. Embrace the journey and discover the joy of walking toward a healthier and happier life.

GOALS/THOUGHTS

> **THE SUN IS THE MOST IMPORTANT THING IN EVERYBODY'S LIFE, WHETHER YOU'RE A PLANT, AN ANIMAL, OR A FISH, AND WE TAKE IT FOR GRANTED.**
>
> — DANNY BOYLE

CHAPTER 14
EMBRACE THE SUN

Disclaimer: Before incorporating any new health practices, including sun exposure, into your routine, it's essential to consult with a healthcare professional, especially if you have any existing health conditions, concerns, or skin sensitivities. While moderate sun exposure can be beneficial for most individuals, each person's needs may vary. This chapter aims to provide general information and recommendations about the benefits of sun exposure but should not replace personalized medical advice.

As we continue our journey towards a "Happy New You!" and a thriving, healthy life, we cannot overlook the importance of the sun's rays and the essential nutrients it provides Vitamin D. Just like plants need sunlight to grow and flourish, our bodies require this vital vitamin to support various bodily functions and overall well-being.

The Power of Vitamin D

Vitamin D is often referred to as the "Sunshine Vitamin" because our bodies can synthesize it when exposed to sunlight. It plays a crucial role in maintaining bone health, supporting the immune system, and regulating mood. Getting enough Vitamin D is essential for overall health and can even help protect against certain chronic diseases.

Harnessing the Sun's Potential

Stepping outside and exposing ourselves to natural sunlight is one of the most effective ways to boost our Vitamin D levels. Spending some time outdoors, especially during the sunnier hours of the day, allows our skin to produce this essential nutrient naturally.

Using DMinder for Optimal Vitamin D Intake

We can use technology to our advantage to make the most of our sun exposure and Vitamin D synthesis. One such tool is the DMinder app, which helps track our Vitamin D production based on factors like location, time of day, and skin type. It assists us in finding the right balance between enjoying the sun and staying safe.

You can find and download the DMinder app for your mobile device by visiting the DMinder App or searching for "DMinder" in your device's app store.

We tend to see the sun as dangerous or just as a Vitamin D liberator, but the sun, especially the morning sun, has many benefits for our health.

Balancing the Body's Circadian Rhythm

Getting morning sunlight helps to kickstart our body's sleep-wake cycle. Getting sunshine into your eyes lights up the brain and sets off a cascade of hormones and neurotransmitters. How amazing is that! It will help get us to sleep at night and wake up easier and more refreshed in the morning. The morning sunlight causes cortisol to be released, which is the wake up hormone, and causes melatonin to be suppressed, the sleep hormone. Getting regular morning sunlight resets this rhythm.

Boost Mood and Mental Health

Getting out into the sun has the benefit of helping people suffering from depression and mental health disorders. Sunlight causes a release of serotonin, helping you to feel happy, positive, and alert. It triggers the release of endorphins, the feel-good hormones. I don't know about you, but seeing the sun out makes me happy.

The sun has amazing qualities that help with our health, but it still has the power to hurt us. You must be smart with sun exposure.

Safety First - Preventing Overexposure

Being mindful of the risks associated with overexposure to the sun is crucial. Prolonged exposure to harmful ultraviolet (UV) rays can lead to sunburn, premature aging, and an increased risk of skin cancer. Here are some safety tips to keep in mind:

Seek Shade: During peak sun hours, typically between 10 a.m. and 2 p.m., seek shade to reduce direct sun exposure.

Wear Protective Clothing: Cover up with loose, long-sleeved clothing and wide-brimmed hats to shield your skin from the sun. Once you have gotten your allotted sun time, you can wear protective clothing to keep from getting burned.

Use Natural SPF: Consider using natural sunscreens with mineral-based ingredients like zinc oxide such as Badger Balm or natural seed oils like raspberry seed, carrot seed and jojoba for added protection. I am not a fan of regular sunscreen as it is full of chemicals that soak into our skin. There are so many natural alternatives that are extremely helpful without being harmful.

Stay Hydrated: Remember to drink plenty of water, especially when spending time outdoors on sunny days. Don't gulp your water, but sip on it throughout the day. Quick overhydration in a short period of time will flush out minerals from your body and can be life-threatening. If you are sweating heavily, an electrolyte powder added to your water will help replace what your are losing from sweating.

Balancing Sun and Safety

Finding the right balance between enjoying the sun's benefits and protecting our skin is essential for overall health and well-being. Embrace the sun in moderation, and be mindful of your body's needs and limits. By using tools like the DMinder app and practicing sun safety, you can optimize your Vitamin D intake while minimizing the risks associated with excessive sun exposure.

By responsibly enjoying the sun's rays, you'll boost your health and cultivate a deeper connection with nature. Embrace the sun with gratitude, and let its warmth and radiance contribute to your journey towards a "Happy New You!"

> THE GRASS IS SOFT! IT'S COOL! I FEEL FREE! RUNNING AROUND IN THE GRASS IN YOUR BARE FEET CAN BE VERY EXCITING...
>
> — CHARLES M. SCHULZ, PEANUTS, 1960 {LUCY & PATTY}

CHAPTER 15
GET GROUNDED - RECONNECTING WITH THE EARTH'S ENERGY

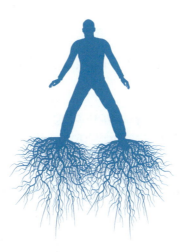

In our fast-paced modern world, we often find ourselves disconnected from the natural world, spending much of our time indoors or walking on a concrete jungle and insulated from the Earth's surface. However, reconnecting with the Earth's energy through the practice of Grounding, also known as Earthing, can offer numerous potential health benefits. In this chapter, we'll explore the concept of grounding, its potential effects, and how you can incorporate this simple yet powerful practice into your daily life.

The Art of Grounding

Grounding involves direct physical contact with the Earth's surface, such as walking barefoot on natural terrain like grass, soil, or sand. The Earth carries a negative electric charge, and through this contact, it is believed that we can absorb electrons from the Earth into our bodies. These electrons are thought to neutralize harmful free radicals and promote balance within the body.

Potential Benefits of Grounding

While the scientific research on grounding is still in its early stages, proponents of the practice suggest a range of potential benefits, including:

Reduced Inflammation: Grounding is believed to have anti-inflammatory effects, which may contribute to easing chronic pain and inflammation.

Improved Sleep Quality: Grounding may help regulate cortisol levels and support healthier circadian rhythms, leading to better sleep.

Stress Reduction: Spending time grounded may promote relaxation and help the body's stress response.

Enhanced Mood: Many individuals report feeling more emotionally balanced and centered after grounding.

Support for the Immune System: Grounding is thought to positively impact the immune system, potentially enhancing its function.

Embracing Grounding in Your Daily Life

Incorporating grounding into your routine is simple and can be a rewarding practice. Here are some ways you can get grounded:

Barefoot Walks: Take advantage of natural surfaces like grass, sand, or soil and walk barefoot. Feel the Earth beneath your feet and allow yourself to reconnect with nature.

Gardening: Engage in gardening or other outdoor activities barefoot so there is direct contact with the Earth.

Nature Time: Spend time outdoors in natural environments. Sit or lie down on the ground and allow yourself to soak in the Earth's energy.

Grounding Products: Consider using grounding mats, sheets, or patches to bring the benefits of grounding indoors, especially during times when going outside may not be feasible.

While many people find grounding to be a positive and transformative practice, it's important to remember that individual experiences may vary. Additionally, while some research supports the potential benefits of grounding, more studies are needed to fully understand its impact on human health.

Reconnecting with the Earth's energy through grounding can be a deeply enriching experience for both mind and body. Whether you choose to walk barefoot on natural terrain, spend time in nature, or utilize grounding products, allow yourself to embrace this simple yet profound practice.

As you get grounded, take moments to breathe in the fresh air and appreciate the beauty of the world around you. Let the Earth's energy nourish and support you on your journey towards a "Happy New You!" May you find peace, balance, and vitality through this ancient practice of grounding.

> "SUCCESS IS THE SUM OF SMALL EFFORTS, REPEATED DAY IN AND DAY OUT."
>
> — ROBERT COLLIER

CHAPTER 16

MASTERING THE BASICS - BUILDING A STRONG FOUNDATION FOR SUCCESS

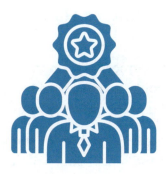

In the pursuit of excellence, one principle stands tall above the rest: mastering the basics and fundamentals. Like a sturdy building that rests on a solid foundation, success is built upon a strong understanding and application of core principles. In this chapter, we'll delve into the wisdom of two remarkable individuals, Coach John Wooden and T. Harv Eker, who both recognized the significance of mastering the basics in their respective fields.

Coach John Wooden: Building Champions from the Ground Up

Coach John Wooden, a revered figure in the world of basketball, understood that greatness was born from a dedication to mastering the fundamentals. He taught his players that they needed to excel at the basics before they could execute complex plays or showcase flashy skills. Dribbling, passing, shooting, and defense were the building blocks for the team's success.

Wooden's coaching philosophy transcended the basketball court and reached into the realm of life itself. He emphasized character development and the importance of building a strong integrity, discipline, and teamwork foundation. Through his famous "Pyramid of Success," he instilled in his players the value of mastering fundamental qualities like industriousness, cooperation, and loyalty.

T. Harv Eker: Learning to Handle What You Already Have

T. Harv Eker, a leading authority on financial success and personal growth, shared a valuable lesson about handling what we already possess. He narrated a poignant story about ice cream.

Picture a bustling park on a beautiful sunny day. Birds chirping, children playing, and the sweet scent of spring in the air. Amidst this, a child relishes a single scoop of velvety ice cream, but as she walks, the yummy scoop plummets to the ground. Heartbreak is evident. Being the doting guardian, you consider a replacement. Yet, as you approach the ice cream truck, she points at the mammoth triple-scoop. Intriguing, isn't it? If the single scoop proved challenging, how could she possibly fare with three?

Eker's rich parable offers a profound truth: Our ability to manage life's complexities is deeply rooted in our command over the basics. Before reaching for more, we must first learn to handle our current resources, be it finances, skills, or opportunities. Building a strong foundation with what we possess lays the groundwork for handling greater responsibilities and abundance in the future.

Embrace the Journey of Mastery

In both sports and life, mastery is not a one-time achievement but a continuous journey of growth and refinement. Just as Coach John Wooden's players practiced their dribbling and shooting daily, we, too must dedicate ourselves to honing our skills, knowledge, and character. The process of mastery demands patience, discipline, and the willingness to start with the basics and progress step by step.

Embrace the simplicity of the journey, for therein lies the magic of transformation. Just as a soaring skyscraper emerges from a well-constructed foundation, your achievements will be a testament to the solid groundwork you lay today.

As we conclude this chapter, remember the wisdom of both Coach John Wooden and T. Harv Eker. The keys to unlocking our full potential are mastering the basics and learning to handle what we have. The foundation you build today will shape your success tomorrow. Stay committed to the journey of mastery, and watch as your dreams take flight upon the strong wings of your unwavering dedication to the fundamentals.

> # NO MATTER HOW SLOW YOU GO, YOU ARE STILL LAPPING EVERYBODY ON THE COUCH,
>
> UNKNOWN

CHAPTER 17
EXERCISE - THE POWER OF STARTING SIMPLE

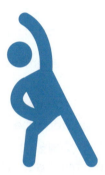

When it comes to transforming our health and well-being, exercise is a key ingredient in the recipe for success. Often, we may feel overwhelmed by the thought of complex workout routines or the need to join a gym. However, the truth is that exercise can start simple, and significant changes can happen right in the comfort of our own homes. In this chapter, we'll explore the world of bodyweight exercises and the remarkable impact they can have on our lives.

The Beauty of Bodyweight Exercises

Bodyweight exercises are a form of strength training that rely solely on the resistance of your own body, eliminating the need for fancy equipment or expensive gym memberships. These exercises utilize natural movements, targeting multiple muscle groups simultaneously, and can be modified to suit all fitness levels.

A Transformative 15 - 30 Minutes

One of the most common misconceptions about exercise is the notion that hours of intense training are required to see results. Even short bursts of regular exercise can be a game changer. By dedicating just 15 - 30 minutes to bodyweight exercises 4 - 5 days a week, you can start experiencing an abundance of benefits:

Improved Strength: Bodyweight exercises engage and challenge your muscles, leading to increased strength and stamina.

Enhanced Flexibility: These exercises promote flexibility and mobility, reducing the risk of injury. When someone has tight muscles, they think they need to stretch, when the majority of the time, their muscles are tight because they are weak. Exercising your muscles and getting stronger has the surprising benefit of increased flexibility. When my back was bad, I had pain and tightness that couldn't be stretched out. Once I became strong, the flexibility returned even without spending that much time stretching.

Weight Management: Regular exercise can support weight management goals by burning calories and boosting resting metabolism.

Mood Elevation: Physical activity releases endorphins, the feel-good hormones, leaving you with a sense of accomplishment and a positive outlook. Exercise is the number one underutilized antidepressant.

Better Sleep: Exercise has been linked to improved sleep quality, aiding in relaxation and restfulness. Just make sure you don't exercise three hours before bed, or it may energize you and keep you from sleeping.

Increased Energy: Regular movement boosts energy levels and combats fatigue.

Start Simple, Start Today

The beauty of bodyweight exercises lies in their simplicity and versatility. You don't need any special equipment; all you need is your own body and a willingness to begin. Here are some simple bodyweight exercises you can incorporate into your routine:

Squats: Stand with your feet shoulder-width apart and squat as if sitting on an imaginary chair. You want to get your butt back like you are going to sit in a dirty outhouse. I know it's not a great visual, but it works. Return to the standing position and repeat.

Push-ups: Place your hands on the floor shoulder-width apart, extend your legs behind you, and lower your chest towards the ground. Push back up to the starting position. If you can't get onto the ground, you can do pushups on the wall or a counter.

Planks: Assume a push-up position, but instead of resting on your hands, rest on your forearms. Keep your body in a straight line and hold the position for as long as you can. Make sure you keep your belly, butt, and legs tight. Push your elbows into the floor to activate your upper back. If you are doing a plank correctly holding everything tight, you will start to shake in seconds. If you can't get onto the floor, you can do a plank on the wall or hold onto a counter. When you contract all muscles, arms, belly, back, butt, and legs, you will feel it and will still get great benefits.

Lunges: Step forward with one leg and lower your body until both knees are at a 90-degree angle; do not let your forward knee go over your toes. Push off the front foot and return to the starting position. Alternate legs.

Remember to Warm Up and Cool Down

Before diving into your bodyweight exercise routine, take a few minutes to warm up your muscles with light cardio exercises like jumping jacks or jogging in place. After your workout, take a moment to cool down with some gentle stretches to prevent muscle soreness and promote flexibility.

The power of exercise lies not in the complexity of the routines but in the consistency of your efforts. You can gradually build strength, endurance, and overall fitness by starting simply with bodyweight exercises. Whether you have 15 minutes or half an hour to spare, invest that time in your well-being and witness the transformative effects it can have on your body and mind. Remember, the journey of a thousand miles begins with a single step. Take that step today, and let exercise catalyze a healthier, happier "Happy New You!"

> **DO NOT SAVE WHAT IS LEFT AFTER SPENDING, BUT SPEND WHAT IS LEFT AFTER SAVING.**
>
> — WARREN BUFFETT

CHAPTER 18
FINANCIAL SUCCESS ON $7 A DAY - UNLEASHING THE 8TH WONDER OF THE WORLD

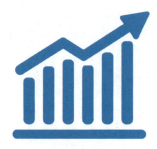

I'm delighted to unveil a powerful strategy that has the potential to transform your financial journey. Combining the wisdom of Chuck Chakrapani's book, "Financial Freedom On $5 A Day," and Bill Staton's book, "The $50 A Month Millionaire," we are taking their proven methods to a whole new level of success.

Life is filled with challenges, but I'm here to guide you toward a path of financial security and abundance. Picture this: with just $7 a day, you can ignite the magic of compound interest and pave the way for lifelong prosperity.

Albert Einstein once referred to compound interest as the "8th wonder of the world," and for a good reason. It's like planting a seed that grows into a mighty oak over time. As your money grows, it earns more money, and that's the magic of compounding.

Now, let's introduce you to The Rule of 72. It's a financial gem that enables you to estimate how long it will take for your investments to double based on your annual rate of return. It's simple yet incredibly powerful.

Have you ever wondered how long it would take for your money to double in an investment? That's where the Rule of 72 comes in - it's like a magic little formula that gives you a quick glimpse into the future of your investments. Simply put, you just divide 72 by your investment's annual return rate. So, let's say you've got a fund that grows at a steady 6% per year. Divide 72 by 6; voila, you'll find it takes roughly 12 years for your money to double. It's that easy!

But here's where it gets really exciting - the Rule of 72 isn't just a neat trick; it's a window into the powerful world of compound interest. Imagine your investment as a snowball rolling down a hill, gathering more snow (or, in this case, interest) as it goes. You're earning interest not only on your original amount but also on the interest already piled up. This snowball effect can turn your investments into a significant sum over time, especially if you're thinking long-term. By understanding the Rule of 72, you're not just crunching numbers; you're unlocking the secret to making your money work for you, giving you a glimpse into how your financial future could unfold.

Imagine channeling your $7 daily into a wise investment, earning a steady 8% annual return. By embracing the power of compound interest, let's see the remarkable journey your savings can embark on:

In just 10 years, your modest $7 daily savings grew to an impressive $39,974. That's quite a leap, isn't it?

Move forward to 20 years, and watch how your dedication boosts your wealth to about $126,276. See how your money is diligently working for you?

Fast forward 30 years, and you've amassed a substantial $312,594. Now, we're entering the realm of significant financial growth.

And finally, after 40 years of consistent saving and the magic of compounding, your commitment blooms into an astounding $714,841! You've not just saved; you've multiplied your wealth beyond the ordinary expectations.

Now, let's expand this vision. Imagine starting this $7 daily investment strategy from day one of a newborn child's life, continuing it all the way until they retire at age 65. This long-term vision can unlock an even more astonishing potential of compound interest. By the time the child reaches retirement age, this consistent, dedicated approach will have grown their savings to an incredible $5,097,296! Starting early, the power of compound interest not only nurtures but dramatically multiplies their savings over the decades, setting a foundation for substantial financial security in their golden years.

This illustration showcases regular investments' incredible potential and compound interest's power over time. It's not just about saving; it's about investing consistently and letting time and interest work their magic on your savings.

Now, I know life is full of distractions and unexpected expenses but remember the wise words of Benjamin Franklin: "Beware of little expenses: a small leak will sink a great ship." So stay mindful of your spending and always prioritize your $7 daily contribution.

With dedication and time on your side, you can transform your financial future. Start now, and watch your wealth grow exponentially with The Rule of 72 as your ally.

I believe in you, and together, we'll unleash the power of compound interest to create lasting financial success. Let's embark on this journey towards prosperity, one step and one $7 investment at a time.

As you dive deeper into Chuck Chakrapani's "Financial Freedom On $5 A Day" and Bill Staton's "The $50 A Month Millionaire," you'll find even more detailed information to help you achieve your financial dreams. This is an investment in your financial education; knowledge is the key to unlocking greater wealth.

Always remember that just like going to the gym to train your muscles, building wealth also requires dedication and consistent effort. You won't see instant results overnight, but with time and commitment, you'll be amazed by how your financial muscles grow stronger.

Together, we can unleash the 8th wonder of the world – compound interest – and set you on a path toward lasting financial success. The journey begins with just $7 a day, and I'm thrilled to witness your transformation into a financially empowered individual.

> **MONEY IS A TOOL. USED PROPERLY IT MAKES SOMETHING BEAUTIFUL; USED WRONG, IT MAKES A MESS!**
>
> — BRADLEY VINSON

CHAPTER 19

THE RICHEST MAN IN BABYLON - BUILDING WEALTH AND EMBRACING FINANCIAL FREEDOM

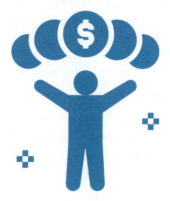

Welcome to the ancient city of Babylon, where the secrets of financial success and wealth were first revealed. In this chapter, we will dive into the timeless wisdom shared in George S. Clason's book, "The Richest Man In Babylon," a treasure trove of financial principles that will transform your financial journey.

At the heart of the book lies a collection of parables set in ancient Babylon, delivering powerful lessons on how to manage your money wisely. As we embark on this journey, let us embrace the spirit of learning and apply the principles to our modern lives.

Start Thy Purse to Fattening: The first tenet urges us to save a portion of our income regularly. Just as a muscle grows with consistent exercise, our wealth grows with regular savings. Cultivate the habit of setting aside a portion of your earnings, even if it's a small amount. Let it accumulate over time, and you'll be astonished by the progress.

Control Thy Expenditures: Wise management of expenses is vital in building wealth. Understand the difference between needs and desires, and prioritize your spending accordingly. Avoid impulse purchases and unnecessary luxuries; instead, invest in assets that will bring lasting value. I have always lived below my means, even when I was in college and had nothing. We are a society of instant gratification and that is how we end up poor, even if we have a very good salary. If I don't have the money for "things," I just don't buy it.

Make Thy Gold Multiply: Putting your savings to work is essential. Invest wisely and let your money grow through various channels such as business ventures, real estate, or long-term investments. Seek advice from experts, study the markets, and be patient with your investments.

Guard Thy Treasures from Loss: Protecting your wealth is as crucial as building it. Avoid risky ventures that promise quick returns but carry significant uncertainty. Diversify your investments and stay informed about potential risks and opportunities. If it sounds too good to be true it is. In the 90's, I had a patient who was in investing and said she could turn 10,000 into 50,000 quickly. I thought that was amazing. My husband didn't see it that way; he saw it as a scam. Well, she ended up going to jail for Ponzi scheme fraud. As I said, if it sounds too good to be true, it is. Be informed and do your due diligence.

Make of Thy Dwelling a Profitable Investment: Homeownership can be a powerful tool for building wealth. Instead of paying rent, consider investing in a property that can appreciate over time and serve as a long-term asset. You may need to give up spending on unnecessary items to be able to save for a house.

Ensure a Future Income: Plan for your future by establishing sources of income that will provide for you and your family in the years to come. Whether it's through investments, retirement plans, or other means, secure your financial well-being.

Increase Thy Ability to Earn: Invest in your knowledge and skills to enhance your earning potential. Continuous learning and personal development open doors to new opportunities and higher income.

Control Thy Expenditure: Revisit this tenet to reinforce the importance of managing expenses wisely. Stay disciplined in your spending habits and avoid unnecessary debt. This one is so important that I put it in twice.

Ensure a Stream of Income for Retirement: Planning for retirement is essential for financial security. Invest in retirement accounts, pension plans, or other vehicles that will provide income when you no longer work.

By understanding and applying the timeless wisdom shared in "The Richest Man In Babylon," you can lay a solid foundation for financial success and embrace the path toward debt-free living. I encourage you to get a copy of the book and study it from cover to cover. Let its teachings become ingrained in your financial psyche, guiding your decisions toward prosperity and abundance.

With every step you take, every dollar you save, and every debt you pay off, you'll be closer to achieving your Happy New You life and lifestyle. Embrace the journey, and let the wisdom of Babylon lead you to a life of financial freedom and fulfillment.

> "SELF-CARE IS HOW YOU TAKE YOUR POWER BACK."
>
> — LALAH DELIA

CHAPTER 20
THE POWER OF MASSAGE FOR YOUR HAPPY NEW YOU

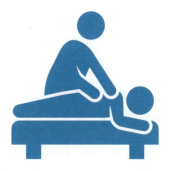

As we continue to explore ways to enhance your well-being, let's dive into the rejuvenating world of massage and discover its incredible benefits.

Many people believe that massage is a luxury or a treat, but I believe it is an essential practice for nurturing both your body and mind. As you embark on this journey of wellness, consider getting several sessions of massage therapy to feel what it is all about. Massage is not just about relaxation; it can be a powerful tool to support your overall health and happiness.

There are three categories of massage therapy: relaxation, therapeutic, and lymph massage. Within those categories are different techniques to get the job done. You may have to try several practitioners to find the one that fits you the best. If you are a person who doesn't like to be touched or doesn't want direct skin to skin contact, there are practitioners that do myofascial release through clothes. There are ways to get the massage that still fit within your comfort level.

Relaxation

Relaxation massage is more general. The therapist will massage all areas of your body, arms, legs, back, and neck. The technique tends to be gentler, allowing you to go into a deep relaxation. I have even fallen asleep in a relaxation massage.

Therapeutic

Therapeutic massage is more focused. The therapist will ask you about your areas of complaint and will focus on them. This is beneficial for sports injuries, work injuries, auto injuries, and chronic areas of pain. Therapeutic massage may be more painful as they work on the areas that are injured or very restricted. Always make sure you let the therapist know if it is too painful, as you don't want to be holding your breath or tightening up if it is too much for your pain level.

Lymph

Lymph massage is a very light technique as the lymph tissue is close to the surface. It would also be considered a relaxation massage, but the goal is different. This massage is highly beneficial for those with edema from cancer, heart issues, and lymphedema. The therapist will massage the entire body to get the lymph draining.

Most people are unaware there is even such a thing as lymph massage. The lymphatic system plays a crucial role in removing waste and toxins from the body, supporting your immune system, and promoting optimal health.

The lymphatic system is like a network of vessels that transports lymph, a fluid rich in white blood cells and waste products, throughout your body. Unlike the circulatory system, which has the heart to pump blood, the lymphatic system relies on muscle movement and external forces like massage to propel lymph fluid.

Lymphatic drainage massage is a specialized technique that involves gentle, rhythmic movements to encourage the flow of lymphatic fluid. By stimulating this system, massage helps to reduce fluid retention, eliminate toxins, and support the body's natural detoxification process.

As you receive a lymphatic drainage massage, you may notice a reduction in swelling and puffiness, particularly in areas prone to fluid retention, such as the ankles, legs, and arms. The improved lymphatic flow also enhances your body's ability to fight infections and boosts your overall immune function.

The many benefits from massage are vast for your physical and mental well-being:

Relieves Muscle Tension: Massage therapy helps to release tight muscles, reduce knots, and alleviate muscular pain. It can improve flexibility and range of motion, making it an excellent option for athletes, and those with physically demanding lifestyles, but it also helps those who are sedentary much of the day.

Eases Stress and Anxiety: Massage triggers the release of endorphins, which are your body's natural feel-good hormones. It promotes relaxation and reduces cortisol levels, helping to combat stress, anxiety, and depression.

Improves Sleep Quality: By promoting relaxation and reducing areas of tension, massage can improve sleep quality and help you fall asleep faster. Adequate rest is essential for your body's rejuvenation and overall well-being.

Enhances Circulation: The rhythmic strokes of massage stimulate blood flow, improving circulation throughout your body. Better circulation ensures that your muscles receive essential nutrients and oxygen, promoting faster healing and recovery.

Boosts Mood and Well-Being: Massage can have a profound impact on your emotional state, leaving you feeling rejuvenated, balanced, and happier. It provides a valuable opportunity for self-care and introspection.

As you incorporate massage into your self-care routine, remember that you are not merely pampering yourself but investing in your physical and mental well-being. Just as you would go to the gym to strengthen your physical body, massage is a vital component of your overall wellness and your journey towards a Happy New You.

So take a moment to relax, breathe deeply, and let the skilled hands of a massage therapist rejuvenate your body and mind. Embrace the power of massage and make it a regular part of your self-care practice. Your Happy New You journey is well on its way, and with the transformative benefits of massage, you'll be closer to achieving your desired state of well-being and contentment.

> THE SPINE IS A LIFELINE. A LOT OF PEOPLE SHOULD GO TO A CHIROPRACTOR BUT THEY DON'T KNOW IT.
>
> — JACK LALANE

CHAPTER 21
DISCOVERING THE POWER OF CHIROPRACTIC CARE

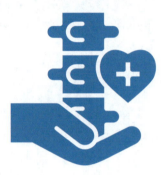

As we continue our quest for a Happy New You, it's essential to explore the incredible world of chiropractic care. I understand you may have heard mixed stories about chiropractors or encountered negative experiences. However, I want you to know that many skilled and caring chiropractors out there genuinely want to help you improve your health and well-being.

Chiropractic care is a holistic approach to wellness that focuses on the relationship between the spine, muscular system, and the nervous system. By making precise adjustments to the spine, chiropractors aim to alleviate pain, improve mobility, and enhance the body's natural healing abilities.

One of the key aspects of chiropractic care is its patient-centered approach. A reputable chiropractor will take the time to listen to your concerns, thoroughly assess your condition, and create a personalized treatment plan that addresses your specific needs and goals.

It's worth noting that chiropractic care is not just for athletes or high-profile individuals. While professional sports teams recognize the value of chiropractic care for their players, it is accessible and beneficial to people from all walks of life.

Regardless of your age, occupation, or activity level, chiropractic care can benefit you in various ways. Whether you're seeking pain relief, improved posture, enhanced mobility, or overall wellness, chiropractic adjustments can be essential to your health journey.

"Look well to the spine for the cause of disease." - Hippocrates

Now, let's explore some of the remarkable benefits of chiropractic care:

Pain Relief: Chiropractic adjustments can help reduce discomfort and pain in various parts of the body, including the back, neck, shoulders, hips, knees, and head. Wherever there is a joint, a chiropractor can work on it.

Improved Mobility: By restoring proper vertebral movement, chiropractic care can enhance your range of motion and flexibility, allowing you to move more freely.

Enhanced Nervous System Function: The spine plays a crucial role in protecting the nervous system. Chiropractic adjustments can ensure that nerve signals flow as freely as possible. Chiropractic care can help with nerve irritation from disc herniations, often preventing the need for surgery.

Preventative Care: Regular chiropractic check-ups can help identify and address potential health issues before they become major concerns, supporting proactive wellness.

Stress Relief: Chiropractic care can help reduce tension and stress in both the body and mind, promoting a sense of relaxation and well-being.

It's essential to find a chiropractor who aligns with your health goals and values. Seek recommendations from friends, family, or trusted healthcare professionals to find a chiropractor who can best meet your needs.

As you embark on this journey of wellness, consider diving deeper into the world of chiropractic care by reading books and articles on the subject. Expanding your knowledge and understanding of this transformative practice can empower you to make informed decisions about your health.

Remember, chiropractic care is about taking a proactive approach to your well-being. It's not just about treating symptoms but addressing the root cause of health issues for long-term improvement.

Unlock the power of chiropractic care on your path to a Happy New You. Embrace the opportunity to experience the wonders of chiropractic adjustments and enhance your overall quality of life.

> "ALMOST EVERYTHING WILL WORK AGAIN IF YOU UNPLUG IT FOR A FEW MINUTES, INCLUDING YOU."
>
> — ANNE LAMOTT

CHAPTER 22
GET UNPLUGGED - EMBRACE NATURE AND DISCONNECT FOR INNER PEACE

In this digital age, we are constantly surrounded by electronic devices that keep us connected and entertained. While technology has brought many conveniences into our lives, it's essential to recognize the value of unplugging from time to time. Getting away from screens and electronic gadgets can have tremendous benefits for our well-being and allow us to reconnect with ourselves and the world around us.

EMFs (Electromagnetic Fields) are a common part of our modern lifestyle, emitted by electronic devices like cell phones, WiFi routers, and computers. While there is ongoing research on the potential health effects of EMFs, it's essential not to approach this subject with fear but with an educational mindset.

Scientists and experts continue to study EMFs to better understand their impact on human health. While some studies show exposure to high levels of EMFs may lead to health issues and oxidative stress, there are other studies that show no health issues. To minimize potential risks, it's a good idea to take simple precautions, like keeping your cell phone away from your body when not in use, using hands-free options, and avoiding excessive exposure. Women, please do not put your phone in your bra, and men, please do not put your phone in your front pocket.

However, instead of focusing solely on EMFs, let's shift our attention to the positive and refreshing benefits of disconnecting from our electronic devices. Stepping away from screens can improve our mental and emotional well-being by reducing stress and anxiety. By immersing ourselves in nature and engaging in outdoor activities, we create opportunities for mindfulness and self-reflection.

Spending time in natural settings, such as parks or nature reserves, can be both rejuvenating and calming. Nature has a way of grounding us and reminding us of life's simple joys. Whether it's a peaceful stroll through a forest, a leisurely hike in the mountains, or a serene moment by the ocean, the natural world offers a powerful antidote to the fast-paced, digital existence we often find ourselves in.

Moreover, engaging in outdoor physical activities can enhance our overall health. Consider joining a walking or hiking group in your community, where you can connect with like-minded individuals while enjoying the beauty of nature. Regular physical activity not only benefits our physical well-being but also contributes to a clearer and more focused mind.

As the day comes to a close, it's essential to recognize the impact of screen time on our sleep quality. The blue light emitted by electronic devices, such as phones and computers, can interfere with our natural sleep-wake cycle and disrupt our ability to fall asleep easily. By unplugging from screens an hour before bedtime and engaging in relaxing activities like reading or meditating, we can prepare our bodies for a restful night's sleep.

Incorporating "unplugged time" into our daily routine can significantly improve our lives. So, challenge yourself to set aside designated moments to disconnect from electronic devices and immerse yourself in the beauty of the world around you. Your mind, body, and soul will thank you.

Remember, we are not advocating for a complete abandonment of technology. Embracing a balanced approach, where we use technology mindfully and allow ourselves moments of disconnection, will lead us to a more fulfilled and harmonious life.

With the world at your fingertips, take the time to get unplugged, venture outside, and discover the simple pleasures that can bring a profound sense of peace and joy to your Happy New You life and lifestyle.

> **KINDNESS IS THE LANGUAGE WHICH THE DEAF CAN HEAR AND THE BLIND CAN SEE.**
>
> ---
>
> MARK TWAIN

CHAPTER 23

THE RIPPLE EFFECT OF KINDNESS - SPREADING JOY ONE ACT AT A TIME

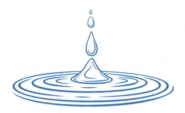

Welcome to a chapter that delves into the profound impact of practicing random acts of kindness and the positive ripple effect it creates in our lives and the lives of others. In a world where negativity sometimes overshadows goodness, we want to remind you of the tremendous power of simple acts of kindness.

Psychological and physiological benefits of kindness

Did you know that when you perform acts of kindness, your brain releases chemicals such as dopamine, serotonin, and endorphins? These natural neurotransmitters are often referred to as the "feel-good" chemicals, and they are associated with pleasure, happiness, and overall well-being. So, not only does doing good make others feel good, but it also boosts your own mood and emotional state.

Besides making you feel good, doing acts of kindness helps to strengthen your immune system, improves energy levels, lowers heart rate and cortisol levels, and improves cognition. Doing acts of kindness helps with depression and anxiety for both the giver and receiver.

Imagine this: You offer a warm smile to a stranger, and their face lights up with genuine happiness. You extend a helping hand to a coworker, and their day is instantly brightened. You surprise a neighbor with a small gift, and they feel deeply appreciated. These moments may seem fleeting, but their impact is profound.

Random acts of kindness create a positive feedback loop. When you perform a kind gesture, it not only brings joy to the recipient but also uplifts your spirit, inspiring you to continue spreading kindness. This positive energy sets off a chain reaction, inspiring others to do the same.

> "Do your little bit of good where you are; it's those little bits of good put together that overwhelm the world."
>
> **Desmond Tutu**

Kindness is contagious

Your act of holding the door for someone may prompt them to do the same for another person, and the ripple effect continues. Small acts of kindness create a domino effect, making the world a brighter and more compassionate place.

So, how can you incorporate more random acts of kindness into your life? It starts with a conscious decision to seek out opportunities to make a positive impact on others. Simple gestures, such as offering a kind word, lending a helping hand, or showing gratitude, can make a world of difference.

Kindness is not limited to grand gestures; it's the everyday actions that matter most. You don't need to change the world all at once. Instead, focus on making someone's day a little brighter with a small act of kindness. The cumulative effect of these actions can lead to significant change.

My brother-in-law was a person who would give the shirt off his back to a stranger. He passed away in 2010, and on his birthday and anniversary my husband and I go to a restaurant and give a tip that is the age he would have been. We have also gone through a drive-through and, given his age, amount to pay for cars behind us. This makes a sad day better. I challenge you to make your hard days into giving days. It will make everyone feel better.

As you make kindness a habit, you'll notice a transformation within yourself. Practicing kindness regularly fosters a sense of fulfillment and joy. The act of giving becomes its own reward, and you'll find yourself seeking out opportunities to bring a smile to someone's face.

Remember that even the smallest acts of kindness can have a lasting impact. Whether it's holding the elevator for a busy colleague or leaving a kind note for a loved one, these gestures create a ripple effect that reaches far beyond their initial occurrence.

So, let's embark on this journey of spreading kindness and joy. Let's be the agents of change, making the world a happier and more compassionate place, one act of kindness at a time. Embrace the ripple effect of kindness, and watch as the world responds with even greater love and positivity.

Together, we can create a world filled with kindness, compassion, and happiness. Let your acts of kindness be the catalyst for a Happy New You and a happier world for all.

Spread the joy and watch it multiply!

> "To forgive is to set a prisoner free and discover that the prisoner was you."
>
> — LEWIS B. SMEDES

CHAPTER 24
THE LIBERATING POWER OF FORGIVENESS - EMBRACE THE GIFT OF RELEASE

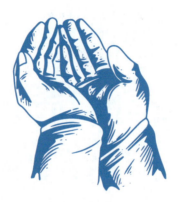

In this transformative chapter, we will explore the incredible power of forgiveness and its profound impact on our lives. Forgiveness is a gift we give ourselves, a powerful tool that liberates our hearts and minds from the burden of past pain and resentment.

Life can present us with challenging and hurtful experiences, and it's natural to feel anger, sadness, or resentment when we are wrong. However, holding onto these negative emotions only keeps us trapped in a cycle of suffering.

Forgiveness is not about condoning the hurtful actions or excusing the wrongdoings of others. It's about freeing ourselves from the heavy weight of grudges and bitterness. When we forgive, we let go of the past, release the negativity, and make room for healing and growth. Forgiveness is for you and not the person you are forgiving.

A beautiful Zen proverb reminds us, "Let go or be dragged." It vividly illustrates that clinging to anger and resentment only leads to prolonged suffering. Instead, when we choose to let go and forgive, we create space for peace and serenity to enter our lives.

Forgiveness is not an instant process, nor is it always easy. It is a journey that requires courage and self-compassion. It's okay to take your time and allow yourself to process the emotions you feel. In this journey of forgiveness, remember that you are not excusing the hurt; you are choosing to release its hold on your heart.

To experience the life-changing power of forgiveness, consider these examples:

Healing Broken Relationships: Forgiveness has the potential to mend broken relationships. When we choose to forgive, we open the door to reconciliation and restoration. It can rebuild trust, deepen connections, and create a stronger bond.

Inner Freedom: Letting go of grudges liberates us from the prison of our own minds. It releases us from replaying past hurts and frees us to fully embrace the present moment.

Emotional Well-Being: Forgiveness contributes to our emotional well-being. By releasing negative emotions, we experience greater peace, reduced anxiety, and improved mental health.

Physical Health: Research has shown that forgiveness is linked to better physical health. It lowers stress levels, strengthens the immune system, and reduces the risk of certain health conditions, such as high blood pressure and cardiac events.

Personal Growth: Forgiveness is a powerful catalyst for personal growth. It allows us to learn from our experiences, develop resilience, and cultivate compassion for ourselves and others.

To begin your journey of forgiveness, start by acknowledging the pain you feel and allowing yourself to grieve. Be gentle with yourself, and remember that forgiveness is a process.

As you practice forgiveness, you may find it helpful to shift your perspective. Try to see the situation from the other person's point of view and recognize that everyone is on their unique journey, influenced by their own experiences and beliefs.

Forgiveness is not about erasing the past, but about rewriting the future. It's about reclaiming your power and choosing love over hate, compassion over resentment, and growth over stagnation.

Embrace the gift of release and experience the profound transformation that forgiveness brings. As you forgive, you create space for new beginnings, inner peace, and a Happy New You.

> "Piglet noticed that even though he had a very small heart, it could hold a rather large amount of gratitude."
>
> — A.A. Milne

CHAPTER 25

THE MAGIC OF THANK YOU CARDS — SPREADING MORE GRATITUDE AND JOY

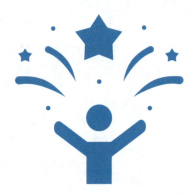

Are you ready to discover a simple yet incredibly powerful way to spread joy and positivity in the world? Get ready to unlock the magic of thank-you cards! These small tokens of gratitude can create a ripple effect of happiness that goes far beyond your expectations.

Imagine this scenario: You had a delightful experience at a cozy little cafe. The barista prepared your coffee just the way you liked it, and the atmosphere felt warm and welcoming. Instead of walking away with a smile on your face, you decide to take it up a notch. You reach into your bag and pull out a charming thank you card.

In the card, you express your heartfelt appreciation for the wonderful service and the delightful coffee. You leave it with the barista, who, later that day, discovers your kind words and thoughtfulness. Instantly, a smile spreads across their face, and their day becomes a little brighter.

But the magic doesn't stop there. The barista, touched by your gesture, decides to pay it forward. They take that positive energy and share it with their co-workers and other customers. Suddenly, the entire cafe is buzzing with a sense of gratitude and happiness. All because of a simple thank you card.

Now, let's explore how you can incorporate this magic into your life

Always be prepared: Keep a stash of thank you cards and stamps on hand. Whether it's in your bag, your desk drawer, or your car's glove compartment, having them readily available means you won't miss any opportunities to spread joy.

Travel with gratitude: When you embark on your journeys, take a few thank you cards along with you. Airlines, hotels, restaurants, and even local tour guides can make your trip memorable. Expressing your appreciation through a thank you card can brighten your day and create a lasting memory.

Acknowledge the everyday heroes: Sometimes, we encounter everyday heroes who make a significant impact on our lives. Maybe it's the bus driver who always greets you with a smile or the friendly neighbor who offers help when you need it. These unsung heroes deserve our gratitude, and a thank you card can show them just how much they are appreciated.

Remember, the act of showing gratitude not only benefits the recipient but also has a profound impact on you. When you take the time to express appreciation, your brain releases dopamine and endorphins—the feel-good chemicals—creating a positive feedback loop. You'll find that as you spread gratitude, you'll also experience a deeper sense of joy and fulfillment.

In the words of a Zen proverb, "A grateful heart is a magnet for miracles." Embrace the magic of thank you cards, and watch as miracles unfold in your life and the lives of those around you. It's the simple yet transformative acts of kindness that can change the world, one thank you card at a time.

> "GROWTH IS PAINFUL. CHANGE IS PAINFUL. BUT NOTHING IS AS PAINFUL AS STAYING STUCK SOMEWHERE YOU DON'T BELONG.
>
> — MANDY HALE"

CHAPTER 26
ALWAYS MOVE FORWARD— EMBRACE PROGRESSION

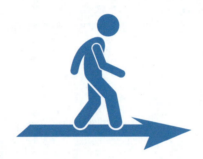

In the game of life, there is no standing still. We are constantly in motion, moving forward or backward. In this chapter, we'll dive deep into the power of always moving forward and embracing the journey of progression.

In the second half of this book, we are reminded that life is a continuous process of growth and evolution. Each step we take, and each decision we make, propels us either toward our dreams or away from them.

Progression is not always about achieving grand milestones or reaching the finish line. It's about the small, consistent steps we take every day to better ourselves and our lives. It is millimeters at a time moving forward. It's about learning from our experiences, embracing change, and constantly evolving.

Just as the seasons change and the tides ebb and flow, life is a dynamic force that demands movement. We must be willing to adapt, to face challenges head-on, and to push past our comfort zones.

Let's celebrate our successes, no matter how small. Let's acknowledge the progress we've made and use it as fuel to keep going. Each step forward, no matter how small, is a victory that deserves recognition.

If we ever stumble or encounter setbacks, let's not view them as failures but as opportunities for growth and learning. Every stumble is a chance to gain strength and resilience, and every setback is a chance to reassess our path and redirect our course.

In the pursuit of a Happy New You life and lifestyle, we must also learn to let go of what no longer serves us. Sometimes, we may need to shed old habits, beliefs, or relationships that hinder our progress. This process of letting go is not easy, but it's necessary for our personal evolution.

Also remember the importance of self-compassion. We are all human, and we all make mistakes. Instead of berating ourselves for our imperfections, let's practice kindness and understanding. Treat yourself as you would a dear friend— with love, patience, and encouragement.

The journey of progression is not always a linear path. It's okay to take detours and explore new avenues. Embrace the adventure of discovery, and don't be afraid to step into the unknown.

Each day presents us with an opportunity to be better than yesterday. Let's approach each morning with gratitude, excitement, and a commitment to make the most of the day ahead.

Let's remember that we hold the pen to our own story. The decisions we make, the actions we take, and the mindset we cultivate shape the narrative of our lives.

Let's be intentional in our choices and bold in our pursuits. Take risks, dream big, and never settle for mediocrity. Life is too short to merely exist; let's live it to the fullest.

Let's continue to support and uplift one another. The power of community and camaraderie is immeasurable. Together, we can achieve so much more than we ever could alone. Find your tribe, the people who love and support you no matter what. They will be essential as you progress on your journey.

Many individuals have faced tremendous adversity and challenges throughout history but chose to keep moving forward. Their stories serve as powerful examples of the indomitable human spirit:

Helen Keller: Despite being deaf and blind from an early age, Helen Keller overcame immense challenges to become a renowned author, political activist, and lecturer. Her unwavering determination and dedication to learning inspired countless people around the world.

Nick Vujicic: Born with a rare disorder called tetra-amelia syndrome, which left him without limbs, Nick Vujicic refused to let his physical limitations define him. He became a motivational speaker and author, spreading a message of hope, self-love, and resilience.

Malala Yousafzai: At just 15 years old, Malala was shot in the head by the Taliban for advocating girls' education in Pakistan. Surviving the attack, she continued her advocacy work, becoming the youngest-ever Nobel Prize laureate for her activism.

These remarkable individuals exemplify the power of determination and the courage to keep moving forward in the face of adversity. They remind us that no matter how challenging life may get, we have the strength within us to rise above and create a life of purpose and fulfillment.

As you embrace the journey of progression, draw inspiration from these stories and know that you, too, have the capacity to overcome obstacles and thrive. Each step you take, no matter how small, brings you closer to the Happy New You life and lifestyle that awaits you.

Remember, you are the architect of your destiny. You have the power to shape your future. So, go forth with confidence, courage, and an unwavering commitment to always move forward. The best is yet to come.

GOALS/THOUGHTS

> **DETOX YOUR MIND, BODY, AND YOUR CONTACT LIST.**
>
> — SUPA NOVA SLOM

CHAPTER 27
DETOXIFY YOUR LIFE— EMBRACE A HEALTHIER AND HAPPIER YOU

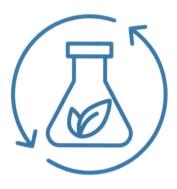

In our pursuit of a Happy New You, it's essential to create a safe and nurturing environment both in our physical spaces and in our social circles. In this chapter, we'll explore the importance of removing toxic elements from our lives, including harmful chemicals and negative people, and how doing so can lead to a more fulfilling and joyous existence.

Effects of toxins on your health

Toxic chemicals are everywhere and are taking a toll on our health. Chemicals that come in contact with our skin may cause itching, redness, rashes, and pain. Chemicals that get ingested can cause abdominal pain, nausea, vomiting, diarrhea, and dehydration. Chemicals that get inhaled may cause drowsiness, dizziness, headaches, confusion, coughing, sinus drainage, blurred vision, and increased heart rate. If you use a chemical and get any of these reactions, even if it is mild, get rid of the product, ASAP.

Eliminating Toxic Chemicals

In our daily lives, we unknowingly expose ourselves to various chemicals present in household cleaners, personal care products, and air fresheners. These toxins can have adverse effects on our health and overall well-being. Many of these products are hormone disrupters and can have an effect on our endocrine system. It's time to make a positive change and opt for natural alternatives that are kinder to our bodies and the environment. If you don't know if your cleaners or personal care products are toxic you can go to the Environmental Working Group website (EWG.org) and look your products up.

Consider switching to natural cleaning solutions like white vinegar and baking soda, which are just as effective in maintaining a clean and sanitary home. Embrace essential oils as a natural way to freshen your living space without harsh chemicals. Additionally, pay attention to the ingredients in personal care products and opt for organic and fragrance-free options to support your health and reduce your environmental impact.

Setting Personal Boundaries with Toxic People

Our social connections play a significant role in shaping our emotional well-being. It's crucial to recognize toxic relationships and create boundaries to protect our mental and emotional health. While it might be challenging, distancing ourselves from negative influences can pave the way for a more positive and fulfilling life.

Identify individuals who consistently bring negativity or drama into your life and assess the impact they have on your overall happiness. Communicate your feelings calmly and assertively, if possible, to them, but be prepared to accept that some toxic people may not change. Remember that setting boundaries is an act of self-care, and it's okay to prioritize your well-being. Setting boundaries can be scary, but it is so important to have them as they create guidelines on how you want to be treated by others. Not having boundaries and giving in all the time will lead to burnout, depression and anxiety.

If you don't fully know how to have boundaries with others there are books available, such as "The Book of Boundaries: Set the Limits That Will Set You Free" by Melissa Urban or "Boundaries" by Drs. Cloud and Thompson that can help you.

Surround Yourself with Positivity

When you remove toxic people from your life, focus on surrounding yourself with positivity and supportive individuals. Seek out like-minded people who uplift and inspire you. Join social groups or communities aligned with your passions and interests to foster meaningful connections and shared experiences.

Practicing Self-Compassion

Embrace self-compassion and understand that it's okay to let go of toxic relationships and situations that no longer serve you. Be gentle with yourself as you navigate this journey towards a happier and healthier you. You deserve love, respect, and positivity in your life.

Letting Go

Zen Proverb wisely states, "Letting go is not giving up. It is the gentle and wise acknowledgment that you can't control another." Releasing toxic relationships is not a sign of weakness; rather, it is an act of empowerment and self-preservation. It opens the door to new possibilities and allows you to welcome positivity and growth into your life.

When you detoxify your surroundings, you create space for personal growth and discover the immense power of self-love and self-respect. Embrace this transformative journey and remember that you hold the key to a happier and healthier you.

Incorporate the wisdom of renowned authors on personal growth and self-care, such as "The Power of Now" by Eckhart Tolle and "The Four Agreements" by Don Miguel Ruiz. Expand your understanding of living a fulfilling life and nurture your well-being on every level.

Remember, you have the strength and resilience to remove toxic elements from your life and embrace a healthier, happier you. As you let go of what no longer serves you, you create space for new opportunities, positive relationships, and a life filled with joy, purpose, and inner peace.

> "CLUTTER IS NOT JUST PHYSICAL STUFF. IT'S OLD IDEAS, TOXIC RELATIONSHIPS, AND BAD HABITS. CLUTTER IS ANYTHING THAT DOES NOT SUPPORT YOUR BETTER SELF."
>
> — ELEANOR BROWNN

CHAPTER 28
EMBRACE THE MINIMALIST LIFESTYLE—DISCOVER THE FREEDOM OF LETTING GO

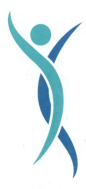

In a world where material possessions often define success, it's easy to accumulate clutter in our homes, cars, and lives. However, deep down, many of us yearn for something more meaningful—a life filled with purpose, freedom, and joy. The minimalist lifestyle offers a path to experience just that.

Minimalism is not about depriving yourself or living with bare essentials. Instead, it's about intentionally letting go of the excess and focusing on what truly matters. By eliminating the unnecessary, you create space to cultivate a life that aligns with your values and passions.

Imagine waking up in a clutter-free home, where every item serves a purpose or brings you joy. Picture stepping into a tidy car that reflects your sense of peace and order. Envision a life free from the weight of material possessions, allowing you to focus on experiences, relationships, and personal growth.

By exploring the minimalist lifestyle, you'll embark on a journey of self-discovery and transformation.

Declutter Your Space

Begin by decluttering one room at a time. Ask yourself if each item brings you joy, serves a purpose, or contributes to your well-being. Donate or sell the things that no longer resonate with you and keep only those that hold significant value.

Detox Your Digital Life

Our digital spaces can also become cluttered with apps, emails, and social media. Unsubscribe from unnecessary newsletters, delete unused apps, and curate your social media feeds to focus on positive and inspiring content.

Prioritize Experiences Over Possessions

Instead of spending money on things, invest in experiences that enrich your life. Travel, attend events, or take up a new hobby. These moments will create lasting memories and bring more fulfillment than any material possession.

Focus on Quality over Quantity

When purchasing new items, prioritize quality over quantity. Invest in items that are built to last and align with your values rather than succumbing to impulse buying.

Practice Gratitude

Embrace gratitude as a daily practice. Be grateful for the things you have and the experiences that shape your life. Gratitude helps shift the focus from what is lacking to the abundance already present.

When you begin to declutter and let go, you'll find that the minimalist lifestyle opens up new possibilities. The more you release, the more space you create for what truly matters. The freedom from the burden of possessions allows you to channel your energy toward personal growth, meaningful connections, and life-enriching experiences. You might even be surprised that you feel more energetic, less depressed, and less anxious when the clutter is gone.

Minimalism is not about perfection but progress. As you take small steps towards simplifying your life, you'll experience a newfound sense of freedom and fulfillment. The minimalist lifestyle empowers you to focus on the essence of life, cherishing each moment and embracing the beauty of living with less.

Remember, exploring minimalism is not about adopting a rigid set of rules. It's about finding what works best for you and embracing a lifestyle that aligns with your aspirations and values.

To deepen your understanding and embark on a transformative journey, consider reading books like "The Minimalist Home" by Joshua Becker and "Goodbye, Things" by Fumio Sasaki. These authors offer valuable insights and practical tips to inspire you on your path to minimalism.

You should open yourself up to the minimalist lifestyle, you'll experience a sense of freedom and lightness like never before. Embrace the art of letting go and discover the richness that comes from living a clutter-free and intentional life. Embrace the minimalist lifestyle, and you'll be one step closer to achieving your Happy New You! Life and lifestyle.

> **FAMILY AND FRIENDS ARE HIDDEN TREASURES, SEEK THEM AND ENJOY THEIR RICHES.**
>
> — WANDA HOPE CARTER

CHAPTER 29
SPEND MORE TIME WITH FAMILY AND FRIENDS—THE POWER OF CONNECTION

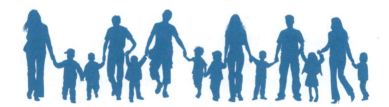

In our fast-paced and digitally driven world, it's easy to get caught up in the hustle and bustle of life, sometimes forgetting the simple yet profound joy of spending time with family and friends. In this chapter, we will explore the importance of nurturing our connections with loved ones and the significant impact it can have on our health and well-being.

Humans are inherently social creatures, and our relationships play a vital role in our overall happiness and fulfillment. Spending quality time with family and friends not only creates cherished memories but also provides numerous health benefits.

Research has shown that meaningful social interactions trigger the release of hormones like oxytocin, often referred to as the "love hormone." Oxytocin fosters a sense of bonding and trust, enhancing our emotional connection with others. Additionally, spending time with loved ones leads to an increase in endorphins and dopamine, the "feel-good" chemicals in our brains, promoting feelings of joy and pleasure.

Even when life gets busy, finding just 15 minutes to connect with a friend or family member over a video call can make a significant difference in both of your lives. Jump on a Zoom or Skype call and enjoy a heartfelt conversation with someone you haven't seen in person for a while. The power of connection is not bound by physical proximity; it transcends space and time.

Creating More Memories

Life is a collection of moments and memories, and spending time with loved ones and good friends allows us to create beautiful and lasting experiences. Whether it's a family gathering, a picnic in the park, or a simple coffee date with a friend, these shared moments become cherished memories that we carry with us throughout our lives.

As the years go by, we may not remember every gift we received or possession we owned, but the memories we create with loved ones stay etched in our hearts forever. Prioritize these moments and make an effort to create more memories with those who mean the most to you.

The Positive Power of Interacting with Others

The positive impact of social connections on our well-being goes beyond just emotional benefits. Numerous studies have shown that individuals with strong social ties have a reduced risk of depression, anxiety, and other mental health issues. Additionally, social interactions can boost our immune system and help us recover faster from illnesses.

Moreover, spending time with friends and family can provide a sense of belonging and purpose. When we share our joys and challenges with others, we build a support network that can help us navigate through life's ups and downs. A strong support system enhances our resilience and ability to cope with stress.

In this digital age, it's easy to get absorbed in virtual interactions and social media. While these platforms can help us stay connected, they cannot fully replace the power of face-to-face or meaningful video interactions. Make an effort to prioritize in-person or video catch-ups, and you'll notice the difference it makes in your life.

So, let's take a moment to reflect on the importance of spending more time with family and friends. It's not just about creating lasting memories or receiving dopamine boosts; it's about building a foundation of love, support, and belonging that enriches every aspect of our lives.

Remember, a simple phone call or video chat can brighten someone's day and deepen your connection with them. Take the time to nurture your relationships, for they are the threads that weave the beautiful tapestry of your life. Embrace the power of connection and experience the profound joy of spending more time with your loved ones.

Explore the joys of spending time with family and friends, you'll find yourself embracing a Happy New You life filled with love, laughter, and meaningful connections.

> "Action is the foundational key to all success."
>
> — PABLO PICASSO

CHAPTER 30
FISH OR CUT BAIT—EMBRACE THE POWER OF TAKING ACTION

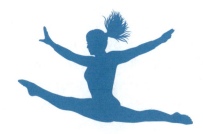

In life, opportunities are like fish in a vast sea, swimming by and presenting themselves in unexpected ways. The question is, are you ready to reel them in, or will you let them slip away? Embracing the power of taking action is like being a skilled angler who knows when to fish and when to cut bait.

It's natural to hesitate and weigh the pros and cons when faced with choices. After all, we want to make the best decisions for ourselves. However, we must be mindful not to overanalyze and let opportunities slip through our fingers. Indecisiveness can leave us stranded on the fence, missing out on the wonders life offers. Do not go into analysis paralysis and do nothing.

The truth is that building the mental muscles to make decisions is a valuable skill. It's like working out at the gym, where every rep strengthens your muscles, making you more capable and resilient. Similarly, every decision you make exercises your mental muscles, making you more adept at facing life's challenges and embracing opportunities.

Embrace Imperfection

Understand that decisions need not always be flawless. Accept that some choices might lead to challenges, but that's where growth lies. Embrace the learning opportunities that come with each decision, whether positive or negative.

Trust Your Instincts

Your gut feeling is often a reliable compass. Our innate instincts may have been suppressed over time, but they remain deeply rooted within us. We have all had a time when we made a decision that was against our gut that didn't turn out right. Learn to trust your intuition, as it can guide you towards the right path.

Visualize Success

Picture yourself thriving after making a decision and taking action. This positive visualization can boost your confidence and encourage you to move forward fearlessly.

Break the Pattern of Overthinking: Recognize when you're spiraling into analysis paralysis. If you find yourself stuck in a loop of overthinking, give yourself a time limit to make the decision. Deep breathing, exercising, or walking can help snap you out of overthinking and can help with making a decision. Sometimes, taking a step forward, even if it feels small, can lead to remarkable breakthroughs.

Embrace a Growth Mindset

Adopt a mindset that perceives challenges as opportunities for growth. With this outlook, you'll welcome decisions as stepping stones towards a more fulfilled life.

Remember, taking action doesn't mean you have to jump into every opportunity that comes your way without thought. It's about being prepared to act when the right moment arrives and trusting yourself to make the best choices for your unique journey.

When you fish, you may not catch every fish you cast for, but each attempt is a step closer to that perfect catch. In the same way, by taking action and making decisions, you'll be moving closer to creating a life filled with exciting possibilities.

As the Zen proverb wisely says, "The journey of a thousand miles begins with a single step."

So, take that first step and embrace the power of taking action. You'll find that the more you build your mental muscles, the more opportunities you seize, and the more fulfilling your Happy New You life will become.

> "It is in your moments of decision that your destiny is shaped."
>
> **Tony Robbins**

> **PEOPLE WILL FORGET WHAT YOU SAID, PEOPLE WILL FORGET WHAT YOU DID, BUT PEOPLE WILL NEVER FORGET HOW YOU MADE THEM FEEL.**
>
> — MAYA ANGELOU

CHAPTER 31
INCREASE YOUR LIKABILITY FACTOR FOR A HAPPIER LIFE

Have you ever noticed how some people seem to effortlessly draw others towards them? Their presence is warm, inviting, and magnetic. This likability factor goes beyond mere charisma; it's an art that anyone can cultivate to enrich their lives and the lives of those around them. In this chapter, we'll explore the power of increasing your likability factor and the numerous benefits it brings to your daily interactions.

Smile, It's Contagious

One of the simplest yet most effective ways to boost your likability is to smile genuinely. A warm smile not only puts others at ease but also releases feel-good neurotransmitters like dopamine and endorphins, making you and others feel happier. By consciously smiling more often, you'll notice a positive shift in your interactions, as people are naturally drawn to those who radiate positivity.

Be a Great Listener

We all love to be heard and understood. Practice active listening by giving your full attention to others during conversations. Show genuine interest in what they have to say, ask thoughtful questions, and avoid interrupting. Being a great listener shows that you value and respect others' opinions, fostering a deeper connection and trust. I have heard that most of us listen only to know what to say next. Next time you are listening, don't listen for what you need to say next; focus on what is actually being said.

Express Sincere Appreciation

Gratitude is a powerful emotion. Expressing genuine appreciation to others for their efforts, kindness, or support can leave a lasting impact. Consider carrying thank you cards and small tokens of appreciation to surprise and uplift those who've made a difference in your life. A little gratitude can go a long way in enhancing your likability and nurturing meaningful relationships.

Show Empathy and Understanding

Put yourself in others' shoes and seek to understand their perspectives and feelings. Demonstrating empathy and compassion creates an environment of emotional safety and trust. By showing genuine concern for others, you'll build stronger connections and be seen as someone who genuinely cares.

Share Positive Energy

Positivity is contagious; those who exude optimism and enthusiasm naturally attract people. Be the source of positive energy in your social circles, uplifting others with your attitude and outlook. Share laughter, offer words of encouragement, and celebrate others' successes. Your uplifting presence will be remembered and cherished by those around you.

Recommended Books to Deepen Your Understanding:

"How to Win Friends and Influence People" by Dale Carnegie: A timeless classic that offers practical advice on building strong and lasting relationships.

"The Like Switch" by Jack Schafer and Marvin Karlins: This book delves into the science of likability and teaches actionable techniques for increasing your social influence.

"The Charisma Myth" by Olivia Fox Cabane: Discover the secrets of charismatic individuals and learn how to enhance your own personal magnetism.

By increasing your likability factor, you'll attract positivity and, enrich your personal relationships and open doors to new opportunities in both your personal and professional life. Like a ripple effect, your likability can create a wave of happiness and fulfillment, making your journey toward a Happy New You even more rewarding.

Remember, genuine likability comes from authenticity and sincerity. Embrace your uniqueness and let your true self shine through your interactions with others. As you continue to cultivate this art of likability, you'll find that life becomes more vibrant, meaningful, and enjoyable, one genuine connection at a time.

> "THE ROOT OF ALL DISAPPOINTMENT IS UNMET EXPECTATIONS.
>
> CHRISTINE HASSLER"

CHAPTER 32
THE POWER OF MANAGING EXPECTATIONS FOR A HAPPY NEW LIFE

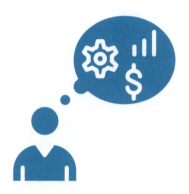

In life's unpredictable dance, curveballs are a guarantee. These unexpected twists often emerge from the actions—or inactions—of people around us. Whether it's friends who don't meet our standards, black swan events that disrupt our routines, or close ones who inadvertently hurt us, such incidents are part and parcel of the human experience. But while we can't control every outcome or every individual, we do wield power over our responses, our expectations, and, by extension, our emotional well-being.

The Weight of Expectations

Each of us carries a set of expectations that shape how we view the world. These unseen scripts influence our reactions to events, situations, and people. While they offer a semblance of predictability, the problem arises when reality doesn't align with our anticipations, ushering in feelings of disappointment, stress, and often heartbreak.

Recognizing the Impact of Unmet Expectations

It's a shared human experience to feel betrayed or hurt when people don't align with our preconceived notions. Over time, these sentiments, if not addressed, can snowball into resentment, leading to fractured relationships and a pervasive sense of dissatisfaction.

However, the silver lining here is the realization that these emotional upheavals often sprout more from our expectations than from others' actions. Recognizing this distinction is the first step to reclaiming emotional balance.

Black Swans, Letdowns, and the Inevitable Unpredictability

Life thrives on unpredictability. Financial hiccups, unforeseen health challenges, or trust breaches by trusted allies—such episodes are not anomalies but rather integral aspects of our existence. The severity of their impact, however, is intimately tied to our expectations. By bracing ourselves for life's inherent uncertainty and accepting the impossibility of perfection, we can better navigate and even find growth in these challenges.

> "Managing expectations is the key to long-term happiness."
>
> **Gary Vaynerchuk**

Crafting a Happy New Life: Tools to Manage Expectations

Self-Reflection and Awareness: Dive deep to discern the origins of your expectations. Are they truly yours or borrowed from society, family, or past experiences? Regular journaling can provide insights and patterns, spotlighting areas needing recalibration.

Embracing Flexibility: Life's essence is its fluidity. Cultivating adaptability ensures that when reality deviates from our scripts, we're not left shattered but rather poised for re-evaluation and growth. None of us are able to control all life events, and the quicker you understand that and adapt to the circumstances, the happier you will be.

Emotional Preparedness: Fortify emotional resilience. Understand that feelings, be they disappointment or elation, are fleeting and don't determine your inherent worth.

Open Conversations: Foster honest dialogues with those who you feel have let you down. More often than not, understanding their viewpoint reshapes our expectations, ensuring they're collaborative rather than unilateral. In the world of technology, it is easy to misunderstand the meaning behind a text or an email. Talking to people in person or on the phone can clarify what they or you meant.

Growth Amidst Disappointment: Every setback conceals a lesson. Instead of ruminating on the disappointment, seek the growth opportunity it presents. My coach and mentor, Mark Edgar Stephens, used to ask me, "What is the blessing?" Trying to find the silver lining in what seems to be an obstacle helps you to focus on the positive. This will keep you moving forward in your journey.

Mindfulness, Meditation, and Gratitude Practice: Stay anchored in the present with mindfulness practices, ensuring external events don't disproportionately sway your emotional equilibrium.

Meditation offers mental clarity, and a daily gratitude practice shifts the focus from what's lacking to what's abundant in your life.

Reaping the Rewards: A Life of Contentment

By mastering our expectations and refining our reactions, we pave the way to genuine contentment. This newfound joy is rooted not in external validations but in the inner alignment of our desires, anticipations, and reactions.

The journey to "Happy New You" isn't about sidestepping disappointments or seeking a life devoid of challenges. It's about equipping ourselves with the tools and mindset to manage, learn from, and even thrive amidst life's inevitable ups and downs. When our happiness springs from within, external events lose their overpowering grip, allowing us to chart a life of joy, contentment, and personal growth.

> I HAVE NOT SEEN ANYONE DYING OF LAUGHTER, BUT I KNOW MILLIONS WHO ARE DYING BECAUSE THEY ARE NOT LAUGHING.
>
> — MADAN KATARIA

CHAPTER 33
THE HEALING POWER OF LAUGHTER—EMBRACE THE JOYFUL SIDE OF LIFE

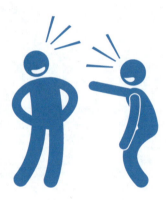

In this chapter, we're going to explore the incredible healing power of laughter and how it can positively impact our physical and emotional well-being. Let's take inspiration from the remarkable journey of Dr. Norman Cousins, who famously laughed his way back to health.

Dr. Norman Cousins was diagnosed with a severe autoimmune disease that left him in excruciating pain. Determined to find a way to alleviate his suffering, he embarked on a journey of self-healing through laughter. Cousins discovered that his pain reduced significantly when he watched funny shows and indulged in hearty laughter. He went on to write the book "Anatomy of an

Illness," which chronicled his experiences and the transformative power of laughter on his health.

Laughter is a natural medicine that can brighten even the darkest of days. When we laugh, our body releases endorphins, which are natural painkillers and mood enhancers. It reduces stress hormones and boosts our immune system, promoting overall well-being. So, let's embrace laughter as a powerful tool in our journey towards a Happy New You.

Tune in to Comedy

Turn off the news and switch on some funny shows or comedy specials. Laughter is contagious, and surrounding yourself with humor can lighten your mood instantly. My husband and I have been scrolling through comedy specials and have found many that make us laugh so hard that our face hurts.

Attend Comedy Clubs

Seek out local comedy clubs and enjoy a night of laughter with friends or loved ones. Live comedy performances have a unique energy that can leave you in stitches.

Discover the Joy of Jokes

Head to your nearest library and pick up a book of jokes. Learning a handful of jokes or riddles can be a fun icebreaker in social situations and bring joy to others. Step 17 in Dr. Richard Schulzes's 20 Steps to A Healthier Life is "Learn 1,000 jokes and laugh."

Now, here's a classic joke to kick-start your laughter:

Why don't scientists trust atoms? Because they make up everything!

Or, what do you call a pig that does karate? A pork chop!

Remember, laughter knows no age, and it's an excellent way to connect with others and spread positivity. Share a laugh with your family, friends, or even strangers you meet along the way. Embrace the power of laughter, and you'll discover that joy has the ability to heal, unite, and uplift us all.

Let's create more laughter in our lives, and as we continue on this journey of self-discovery, may our laughter be our constant companion, guiding us toward a happier and healthier life.

> "CULTIVATE THE HABIT OF BEING GRATEFUL FOR EVERY GOOD THING THAT COMES TO YOU, AND TO GIVE THANKS CONTINUOUSLY. AND BECAUSE ALL THINGS HAVE CONTRIBUTED TO YOUR ADVANCEMENT, YOU SHOULD INCLUDE ALL THINGS IN YOUR GRATITUDE."
>
> — RALPH WALDO EMERSON

CHAPTER 34

THE ART OF GRATITUDE— EMBRACE THE POWER OF MAYBE YES, MAYBE NO

In this chapter, we'll explore the profound concept of gratitude and the transformative practice of appreciating the moments of "Maybe Yes, Maybe No" in our lives, drawing inspiration from a Zen story that reminds us of the beauty of uncertainty.

In a small village, there lived an old farmer. He had a magnificent horse that the villagers admired greatly. One day, the horse managed to escape from the stable, and the villagers rushed to console the farmer, saying, "What a terrible misfortune! Your precious horse is gone!"

To their surprise, the old farmer calmly replied, "Maybe yes, maybe no."

A few days later, the horse returned to the village, leading a wild herd of horses back to the farmer's stable. The villagers congratulated him, saying, "What incredible luck! You are now a wealthy man with all these horses!"

Again, the old farmer replied, "Maybe yes, maybe no."

As days passed, the farmer's son attempted to tame one of the wild horses. However, the horse threw him off and broke his leg. The villagers rushed to console the farmer, saying, "How unfortunate! Your son's leg is broken, and now he cannot help you with the farm work."

Once again, the old farmer replied, "Maybe yes, maybe no."

A few weeks later, the kingdom went to war, and all the young men in the village were conscripted into the army. The farmer's son was spared due to his broken leg. The villagers marveled at the farmer's good fortune, saying, "You are truly blessed; your son is safe from the horrors of war!"

With a serene smile, the old farmer replied, "Maybe yes, maybe no."

This Zen story teaches us the power of embracing uncertainty and being grateful for each moment, even if it may seem unfavorable at first. It reminds us that life is a beautiful dance of "maybe yes, maybe no," and there is much to appreciate in the ebb and flow of experiences.

Gratitude is a practice that can open our hearts and minds to the abundance of life. It allows us to see the silver lining in challenging situations and find joy in the simplest pleasures. By cultivating gratitude, we shift our focus from what we lack to what we have, creating a positive ripple effect in our lives.

Gratitude Journal

Dedicate a few minutes each day to write down three things you are grateful for. If you keep coming up with the same three things or it doesn't feel genuine, then ask yourself, "What three things went well today?" This will make your brain focus on the positives of your day. This simple act can bring immense joy and perspective to your life.

Mindful Moments

Pause and appreciate the beauty around you—the warmth of the sun, the sound of birds chirping, or the smile of a loved one. When in nature, practice Forest Bathing. Don't just go into nature to exercise, but take the time to really focus on the natural world around you; feel it, smell it, experience it.

Acts of Kindness

Practice random acts of kindness and express your appreciation to others. Small gestures can have a big impact. My husband is the king of acts of kindness. He is always doing something kind for someone, whether it is bringing donuts, sending a nice card, or buying flowers for someone. He routinely makes people's day.

The Gift of Presence

Be fully present in the moments you share with others. Listen attentively and savor the connections you make. A person who listens only to formulate their next response, rather than genuinely engaging with the speaker's message, can be described as "waiting to talk" rather than actively listening. Practice listening without trying to figure out what you want to say next.

When we embrace gratitude and the wisdom of "maybe yes, maybe no," we can cultivate a sense of contentment and joy in our lives. Let's journey with open hearts and appreciative spirits, for in each moment, we find the magic of life's unfolding.

> **THE TIME TO RELAX IS WHEN YOU DON'T HAVE TIME FOR IT.**
>
> — SYDNEY J. HARRIS

CHAPTER 35

THE POWER OF RELAXATION— EMBRACE THE ART OF LETTING GO

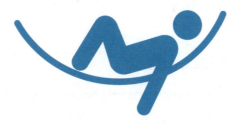

In the hustle and bustle of modern life, we often find ourselves racing against the clock, juggling multiple responsibilities, and striving to stay in control of everything. We wear our busyness like a badge of honor, as if being in a constant state of motion is a sign of success. But in this perpetual cycle of doing, we often forget the art of simply being.

Amidst the chaos, we yearn for moments of peace and tranquility—those rare instances when time seems to slow down, and we can breathe freely without the weight of the world on our shoulders. These are the moments of relaxation, the antidote to stress, and the gateway to a healthier, more balanced life.

As we journey towards our Happy New You, it's essential to recognize the immense power of relaxation and the impact it has on our physical, mental, and emotional wellbeing. It's not merely a luxury or a fleeting indulgence; rather, relaxation is a fundamental necessity for a harmonious and fulfilling life.

So, how can we embrace the art of letting go and incorporate relaxation into our daily lives?

Embrace the Present Moment

The practice of mindfulness invites us to be fully present in each passing moment. By letting go of thoughts about the past or anxieties about the future, we can immerse ourselves in the beauty of the present. Mindfulness techniques such as meditation and deep breathing can help center our minds and bring us back to the here and now.

Unplug and Disconnect

In the digital age, we are constantly bombarded with notifications, updates, and information. Taking time to unplug from electronic devices and social media is essential for recharging our minds and reconnecting with ourselves. Designate specific periods each day for a digital detox, allowing your mind to rest and recalibrate. Turning off electronics an hour before bed helps the brain to unwind.

Nature's Therapy

Nature has a unique way of soothing our souls and restoring our sense of wonder. Whether it's a leisurely stroll in the park, a hike in the mountains, or a day at the beach, immersing ourselves in natural surroundings can have a profound calming and grounding effect. Something so easy as taking your shoes off and walking in your yard for several minutes could have a profound effect.

The Joy of Creative Expression

Engaging in creative activities can be incredibly therapeutic. Whether you enjoy painting, writing, playing a musical instrument, or crafting, creative expression provides an outlet for emotions and fosters a sense of accomplishment and relaxation.

Practice Yoga or Tai Chi

Both yoga and tai chi are ancient practices that combine movement and mindfulness. These gentle exercises promote relaxation, flexibility, and mental clarity, helping us release tension and find balance in our lives.

Soothing Self-Care Rituals

Pampering ourselves with self-care rituals is not self-indulgence but an act of self-love. Taking a warm bath with essential oils, indulging in a massage, or savoring a cup of herbal tea while reading a book are simple yet profound acts of self-care that can alleviate stress and promote relaxation.

Cultivate Gratitude

Like we explored in Chapter 30, gratitude is a powerful practice that fosters relaxation and contentment. By taking time each day to express gratitude for the blessings in our lives, we shift our perspective and invite positivity into our hearts.

In our pursuit of relaxation, it's crucial to let go of the need to control everything. We must recognize that control is an illusion and that we cannot dictate every aspect of our lives. Instead, we should embrace the art of surrender, finding comfort in knowing that not everything needs to be controlled.

By carving out time for relaxation each day, we replenish our inner reserves and gain the clarity and energy needed to face life's challenges with a fresh perspective. As we let go of the need to control, we free ourselves from unnecessary burdens, allowing us to live more authentically and joyfully.

So, make relaxation a priority in your life. Whether it's a few moments of deep breathing during a busy day or a more extended session of creative expression, embrace the art of letting go. By doing so, you'll discover a newfound sense of peace and well-being that will ripple through every aspect of your life. Remember, in these moments of relaxation, we truly find ourselves and experience the essence of a Happy New You.

When we venture into the second half of our journey together, let relaxation become your constant companion—a guiding light amidst the chaos and a source of rejuvenation for your mind, body, and soul. Here's to a life filled with relaxation and the wisdom to cherish each moment of restful bliss.

> "Just be and enjoy this moment. Let go of the illusion of control and embrace the art of relaxation. There is profound power in letting go."
>
> **Unknown**

Remember, each small moment of relaxation is a gift to yourself and a step towards a happier, healthier, and more fulfilled life. So, take a deep breath, release the tension, and welcome the serenity of the present moment. As you do so, you'll find that relaxation is not merely an escape from the demands of life but a profound way of nourishing your mind, body, and soul. Let go and embrace the art of relaxation as you continue your journey towards a Happy New You.

> **STANDING IS BETTER THAN SITTING, MOVING IS BETTER THAN STANDING.**
>
> — JOAN VERNIKOS

CHAPTER 36

SITTING IS THE NEW SMOKING— RECLAIM YOUR HEALTH AND VITALITY

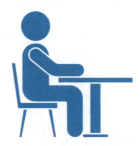

In today's fast-paced world, many of us find ourselves bound to our chairs, desks, or couches, indulging in hours of sitting without realizing the profound impact it can have on our health. Just like we thought with smoking early on, the seemingly harmless act of sitting for extended periods has become a silent health hazard, affecting millions of lives worldwide. In this chapter, we'll delve into the detrimental effects of prolonged sitting and unveil three essential steps to break free from this sedentary trap.

The Perils of Prolonged Sitting

We've become more engrossed in our modern lifestyle, the prevalence of sedentary behavior has skyrocketed, leading to numerous health risks.

Physical Health Hazards

Research has unveiled that prolonged sitting is associated with an increased risk of heart disease, type 2 diabetes, obesity, digestive issues, and certain cancers. A lack of physical activity negatively impacts our metabolism, leading to weight gain and escalating the chances of chronic illnesses. Prolonged sitting will also increase your risk of high blood pressure.

Muscular Imbalances

Prolonged sitting can lead to various muscular imbalances. The most common issue is a weakening of the muscles that support proper posture, such as the erector spinae and core muscles, leading to slouched shoulders and a curved spine. Simultaneously, sitting can overwork the hip flexors, causing them to tighten and potentially leading to lower back pain. Additionally, extended sitting can weaken gluteal muscles, which play a crucial role in hip and lower back stabilization. There is no reason for our core and glutes to be active while sitting; over time, they start to weaken. The term glute amnesia has been coined for those who prolonged sit and the glutes start to shut down.

Impaired Circulation

Sitting for prolonged periods hinders blood flow and circulation, causing blood to pool in the feet. Prolonged sitting increases your risk of not just swollen ankles but more severe conditions like blood clots and varicose veins.

Mental Well-being Impact

The sedentary lifestyle also takes a toll on our mental health. Sitting for extended periods is linked to increased stress, anxiety, and even depression, affecting our overall well-being.

Taking Action to Regain Your Vitality

Breaking free from the sitting trap requires a commitment to reclaiming your health and embracing an active lifestyle. Here are three essential steps to get you started on your journey to vitality.

Move Regularly

Incorporate movement breaks into your daily routine. Set a timer to remind yourself to stand up and stretch, walk around, or do a few simple exercises every hour. Stand and move around when you have a phone meeting. These short bursts of movement can work wonders for your overall health and help counteract the negative effects of sitting.

Engage in Regular Exercise

Make physical activity an integral part of your daily life. Whether walking, jogging, cycling, swimming, or practicing yoga, find activities you enjoy and can easily incorporate into your schedule. Aim for at least 30 minutes of moderate-intensity exercise most days of the week.

Embrace Active Habits

Seek opportunities to stay active throughout the day. Opt for the stairs instead of the elevator, park farther away from your destination to get some extra steps in, or take walking breaks during your lunch hour. Small changes in your daily routine can make a significant difference in combating the sedentary lifestyle.

Remember, you have the power to break free from the sedentary lifestyle. Taking action and prioritizing movement and physical activity can reclaim your health, boost your energy, and improve your overall well-being.

In the next chapter, we'll introduce you to the incredible practice of hanging, which complements your efforts to combat the negative impacts of sitting. So, stay tuned for more insights on how to unleash your full potential for a Happy New You life and lifestyle!

> "OUR BODIES ARE DESIGNED FOR MOVEMENT, NOT STAGNATION. HANGING PULLS US OUT OF OUR SEDENTARY HABITS AND BACK INTO ALIGNMENT WITH OUR NATURE."
>
> — GRAY COOK, PT

CHAPTER 37

HANG YOUR WAY TO A HEALTHIER SPINE AND STRONGER GRIP

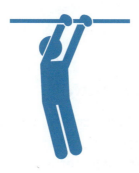

In our quest for a Happy New You, we often seek out ways to improve our physical well-being and overall health. One often overlooked yet incredibly effective practice is hanging—a simple but powerful way to boost spinal health and grip strength. Whether you choose to hang from a chin-up bar or use an inversion table, both methods offer an array of benefits that can greatly impact your well-being. In this chapter, we'll dive into the advantages of hanging, backed by research and studies, and explore how this practice can contribute to your journey of self-improvement.

There are many health benefits for hanging and inverting.

Decompression of the Spine

The constant downward force of gravity compresses our spinal discs throughout the day. Hanging from a bar or an inversion table allows for decompression, creating space between the vertebrae and promoting better spinal alignment and health. This natural traction can relieve pressure on nerves and reduce discomfort caused by conditions like sciatica or lower back pain.

Improved Flexibility

Hanging stretches, the spine and surrounding muscles, promoting flexibility and mobility. It can be especially beneficial for individuals with sedentary lifestyles or those who spend long hours sitting at a desk, counteracting the negative effects of a static posture.

Enhanced Core Strength

Maintaining stability while hanging engages the core muscles, including the abdominals and obliques. Over time, this can lead to improved core strength and better support for your spine during daily activities.

Strengthening Forearm and hand Muscles

When you hang from a bar or other suspended structure, your fingers, hands, and forearms must engage to support your body weight. This strengthens the muscles responsible for gripping and enhances the stability of your wrists and shoulders.

Injury Prevention

Strong grip strength can help prevent injuries related to the hands and wrists, as it provides better support and stability during physical tasks.

Scientific Studies on Hanging

A study published in the Journal of Physical Therapy Science found that inversion table therapy effectively reduced lumbar pain and improved functional status in patients with chronic low back pain. The research highlighted the potential of inversion therapy as a non-invasive and safe method for managing back pain.

Another study published in the Journal of Clinical Rehabilitation revealed that regular hanging exercises improved grip strength and forearm endurance in healthy individuals. The researchers concluded that hanging exercises could be a simple and accessible way to enhance grip strength and forearm function.

"Think of hanging as an antidote to the modern life of sitting and slouching. It's not just exercise; it is a return to functional movement, essential for our spine and overall health."—Katy Bowman.

Incorporating Hanging into Your Routine

Chin-Up Bar Hanging

Find a sturdy chin-up bar at your gym or invest in a doorway pull up bar for home use. Start with shorter hanging sessions and gradually increase the duration as you build strength and tolerance. Don't worry if you can't hang for more than a few seconds. This is a process, and you will improve over time. Aim for daily or semi-daily sessions, incorporating them into your warm-up or cool-down routines.

Inversion Table Therapy

If you prefer a more controlled inversion experience, consider using an inversion table. Consult a healthcare professional or therapist if you have any pre-existing health conditions or concerns. Follow the manufacturer's instructions and ensure that the table is properly adjusted to your height and comfort.

Remember to approach hanging exercises with care and listen to your body. If you experience discomfort or pain, discontinue the practice and seek advice from a qualified healthcare professional.

When you hang your way to a healthier spine and stronger grip, you'll be nurturing your body and taking another positive step on your journey to a Happy New You. Embrace this effective and accessible practice, and witness the incredible benefits it can bring to your overall well-being.

> "INSPIRATION EXISTS, BUT IT HAS TO FIND YOU WORKING."
>
> — PABLO PICASSO

CHAPTER 38
UNLEASHING YOUR CREATIVE POTENTIAL—EMBRACE THE POWER OF IMAGINATION

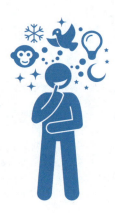

In today's fast-paced and structured world, we often overlook the immense power of our creative minds. Yet, creativity is not limited to artists and musicians alone; it's an inherent trait within each one of us. Embracing and nurturing our creative potential can lead to greater happiness, fulfillment, and a more vibrant life. In this chapter, we will explore the importance of unleashing our creative potential, the positive impact it has on various aspects of our lives, and practical steps to tap into our boundless imagination.

The Power of Creativity: A Comprehensive Exploration

Expression of Authenticity

Creativity is a unique expression of our authentic selves. When we engage in creative pursuits, we connect with our inner voice and express our thoughts, feelings, and experiences in ways that words alone cannot capture. For example, consider Frida Kahlo's paintings, which vividly express her pain and resilience, offering a glimpse into her soul that words could never fully convey. This authenticity resonates deeply with others, creating a powerful connection.

Enhancing Problem-Solving Skills

Creativity goes hand in hand with problem-solving. When we approach challenges with a creative mindset, we open ourselves up to innovative and unconventional solutions. Thomas Edison famously said, "I have not failed. I've just found 10,000 ways that won't work," highlighting how creativity fosters persistence and breakthrough solutions. Whether in personal life or professional endeavors, a creative approach can transform obstacles into opportunities for growth.

Stress Reduction and Mental Health Benefits

Engaging in creative activities can be incredibly therapeutic and serve as a form of stress relief. Studies show that activities like painting, drawing, and writing can significantly reduce cortisol levels, the body's primary stress hormone. By immersing ourselves in the creative process, we quiet the noise of the outside world, promoting a sense of calm and mindfulness. Art therapy, for example, is used to help individuals cope with trauma, anxiety, and depression by allowing them to express themselves in a non-verbal medium.

Boosting Self-Confidence

As we explore and develop our creative talents, we gain a sense of achievement and increased self-confidence. The act of creating something from scratch and seeing it come to life empowers us to believe in our abilities and potential. For instance, a novice baker who successfully makes a cake from scratch gains confidence not only in baking but also in other areas of life. This newfound self-assurance can have a ripple effect, enhancing our overall sense of self-worth and competence.

Fostering Connection and Community

Creativity is a universal language that bridges gaps and connects people from different backgrounds and cultures. Engaging in creative activities can strengthen relationships and foster a sense of community and understanding. Community art projects, like mural painting, often bring neighborhoods together, creating bonds and shared pride. Events such as local art fairs, music festivals, and writing workshops provide opportunities for individuals to connect over shared passions and creative expressions.

Practical Steps to Unleash Your Creative Potential

Embrace Curiosity

Curiosity is the spark that ignites creativity. Allow yourself to be curious about the world around you, explore new ideas, and ask questions. Approach life with childlike wonder and an open mind, ready to absorb inspiration from the smallest of details. Albert Einstein once said, "The important thing is not to stop questioning. Curiosity has its own reason for existing." By nurturing curiosity, we open ourselves up to endless possibilities and creative ideas.

Cultivate Playfulness

Creativity thrives in a playful environment. Give yourself permission to play, experiment, and make mistakes. Let go of self-judgment and embrace the process of exploration without the fear of being perfect. Remember, some of the greatest inventions, like the Post-it Note, were the result of playful experimentation and unexpected outcomes. Embracing a playful attitude encourages risk-taking and innovation, essential components of the creative process.

Create a Creative Space

Designate a specific area in your home or workspace as a creative sanctuary. Fill it with materials and tools that inspire you, such as art supplies, musical instruments, or writing utensils. Having a dedicated space will encourage you to spend time being creative. Consider the example of Virginia Woolf, who emphasized the importance of having "a room of one's own" for creative work. This space becomes a haven for imagination and productivity.

Engage in Diverse Activities

Try various creative pursuits to discover what resonates with you the most. Experiment with painting, writing, photography, dancing, cooking, or any other activity that sparks your interest. You might find unexpected joy in exploring new talents. For instance, actor and martial artist Bruce Lee found peace and creativity in writing poetry. Engaging in diverse activities broadens our creative horizons and enriches our skill set.

Set Aside Time for Creativity

Life can get busy, but carving out time for creative pursuits is essential. Whether it's a few minutes each day or a dedicated weekend, prioritize creative time to nourish your mind and soul. Renowned author Haruki Murakami dedicates several hours each morning to writing, demonstrating the power of a consistent creative routine. Scheduling regular creative sessions helps integrate creativity into our daily lives.

Seek Inspiration

Surround yourself with inspiration. Attend art exhibitions, read books, watch films, listen to music, and immerse yourself in nature. Inspiration is everywhere, waiting to awaken your creativity. For example, Steve Jobs often cited his calligraphy class as a major source of inspiration for the design of Apple products. By exposing ourselves to diverse sources of inspiration, we stimulate our creative minds and generate new ideas.

Embrace Failure as Growth

Not every creative endeavor will result in a masterpiece, and that's perfectly okay. Embrace failure as part of the learning process and an opportunity for growth. Each experience contributes to your creative journey. Remember, J.K. Rowling's "Harry Potter" manuscript was rejected by 12 publishers before becoming a global phenomenon. Viewing failure as a stepping stone rather than a setback empowers us to persist and evolve creatively.

> "Logic will get you from A to B. Imagination will take you everywhere."
>
> **Albert Einstein**

Unleashing your creative potential is a powerful step towards a Happy New You. Embrace the magic of your imagination, and you'll find that creativity opens up new possibilities, fuels your passions, and infuses every aspect of your life with joy and purpose.

GOALS/THOUGHTS

> **THE OAK FOUGHT THE WIND AND WAS BROKEN, THE WILLOW BENT WHEN IT MUST AND SURVIVED.**
>
> — ROBERT JORDAN

CHAPTER 39

CULTIVATING RESILIENCE— BOUNCING BACK STRONGER THAN EVER

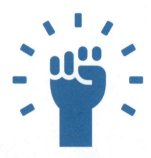

Life is full of ups and downs, challenges, and setbacks. Cultivating resilience is a vital skill that can help us navigate through difficult times with grace and strength. In this chapter, we will delve into the power of resilience and discover how it can empower us to bounce back stronger than ever before. Let's explore the key components of resilience and learn practical strategies to enhance this invaluable trait in our journey to a Happy New You.

Understanding Resilience

Resilience is more than just bouncing back from adversity; it's the ability to adapt and thrive in the face of challenges. Here are the key components of resilience:

Adaptability

Resilience involves the ability to adapt and adjust to changing circumstances. It's about being flexible in the face of challenges and finding alternative paths when the original one is obstructed.

Positive Mindset

Resilient individuals tend to maintain a positive outlook even in challenging situations. They focus on solutions rather than dwelling on problems, fostering a sense of hope and optimism.

Emotional Regulation

Resilience includes the capacity to manage and regulate emotions effectively. It's about acknowledging and processing emotions without being overwhelmed by them.

Social Support

Strong social connections play a crucial role in resilience. Having a support system of family, friends, or community can provide comfort and encouragement during tough times.

Growth Mindset

Resilience is closely linked to a growth mindset, the belief that challenges are opportunities for growth and learning. Embracing setbacks as stepping stones to progress fuels resilience.

Cultivating Resilience:

Build Emotional Awareness

Practice self-reflection and emotional awareness to understand your reactions to adversity. Cultivate mindfulness and meditation to better manage stress and emotions.

Reframe Challenges

Train your mind to reframe challenges as opportunities for growth and learning. Focus on the lessons and insights gained from difficult experiences.

Seek Support

Reach out to trusted friends, family members, or support groups during tough times. Having someone to listen and empathize with you can make a significant difference.

Strengthen Coping Skills

Develop healthy coping mechanisms to manage stress and anxiety. Engage in activities that bring joy and relaxation, such as hobbies, exercise, or creative outlets.

Foster Resilience Through Mindfulness

Practice mindfulness to build resilience by staying present, non-judgmental, and accepting of your emotions and circumstances.

Real-Life Resilience Story:

Meet Sarah (not her real name, a former patient of mine), a remarkable woman who demonstrated extraordinary resilience in the face of adversity. At the age of 30, Sarah was diagnosed with a life-threatening illness that changed her world overnight. As she navigated through the challenging journey of treatments, surgeries, and emotional turmoil, Sarah's resilience shone brightly.

The initial shock of the diagnosis left Sarah feeling overwhelmed and fearful of the uncertain future. However, with the support of her family, friends, and medical professionals, she slowly learned to accept her new reality. Instead of succumbing to despair, Sarah adopted a growth mindset, believing she could find meaning and purpose even in difficult circumstances.

Throughout her treatment, Sarah made a conscious effort to build emotional awareness. She allowed herself to feel full emotions, from anger and sadness to hope and gratitude. Through mindfulness and meditation, she learned to let go of anxieties about the future and stay present in each moment, cherishing the joys that life still had to offer.

Sarah's resilience also relied on her ability to reframe challenges. Instead of dwelling on what she had lost, she focused on what she had gained—a newfound appreciation for life, a deep connection with loved ones, and the strength to face adversity head-on. Sarah began to view her illness as an opportunity for personal growth and transformation.

While the road to recovery was long and arduous, Sarah's unwavering determination and support system helped her overcome obstacles one step at a time. She embraced her vulnerability and allowed herself to lean on others when needed, finding solace in their love and care.

As Sarah emerged from the depths of her illness, she became a source of inspiration for others facing similar challenges. Through her journey, she found her purpose in helping others cultivate resilience and embrace life with courage and gratitude.

In the words of Albert Einstein, "Adversity introduces a man to himself." Sarah's journey exemplified the power of resilience, proving that even in the darkest of times, we can find strength within ourselves to rise above adversity and embrace life with renewed vigor.

As we embark on our journey to a Happy New You, let us draw inspiration from Sarah's story and cultivate resilience. May we face life's challenges with courage, positivity, and a growth mindset, knowing that we have the power to bounce back stronger than ever before.

> "THE MOST TERRIFYING THING IS TO ACCEPT ONESELF COMPLETELY."
>
> CARL JUNG

CHAPTER 40

NURTURING SELF-COMPASSION—EMBRACE YOUR IMPERFECTIONS

In the pursuit of a Happy New You, it's essential to cultivate self-compassion. This chapter delves into the power of self-compassion and its role in fostering well-being, resilience, and a positive outlook on life. Let's explore what self-compassion truly means, why it's important, and practical ways to nurture this transformative trait.

The Essence of Self-Compassion

Self-compassion is the act of treating ourselves with the same kindness, understanding, and support that we would offer to a dear friend. It involves acknowledging our imperfections, accepting them, and embracing our humanness with warmth and empathy. Unlike self-esteem, which can be contingent on achievements or external validation, self-compassion is unconditional and doesn't require us to be perfect or flawless.

Overcoming Self-Criticism

We often engage in self-criticism, focusing on our mistakes and flaws. This self-criticism can be detrimental to our well-being and lead to feelings of inadequacy and unworthiness. Self-compassion offers an alternative, encouraging us to be kind and understanding toward ourselves, even when we fall short.

Building Resilience

Self-compassion acts as a buffer during difficult times, providing comfort and support when facing challenges. Instead of being overly self-critical or judgmental, self-compassion helps us navigate through tough moments with greater ease and bounce back stronger.

Enhancing Mental Health

Embracing self-compassion fosters a healthier relationship with ourselves and decreases negative self-talk. It can reduce symptoms of anxiety, depression, and stress, promoting a more positive outlook on life.

> "Owning our story and loving ourselves through that process is the bravest thing that we will ever do."
>
> **Brené Brown**

Practical Ways to Cultivate Self-Compassion:

Mindful Self-Awareness

Practice mindfulness to become aware of your inner dialogue and self-critical thoughts. When you catch yourself being harsh or judgmental, gently redirect your thoughts toward self-compassion.

Treat Yourself Like a Friend

Imagine how you would respond to a friend facing a similar situation. Offer yourself the same care and encouragement you would extend to them. We are often kind to others who don't deserve it but are horrible to ourselves. It is time to treat ourselves with kindness, compassion, and love.

Embrace Imperfection

Recognize that perfection is unattainable and that everyone makes mistakes. Embrace your imperfections as a part of being human and an opportunity for growth. No one is perfect, and trying to be perfect only creates stress and anxiety.

Practice Self-Kindness

Be compassionate toward yourself in moments of difficulty or failure. Treat yourself with kindness, as you would care for a loved one going through a challenging time. Beating yourself up only makes things worse. Be kind.

Release Unrealistic Expectations

Let go of unrealistic expectations and self-imposed standards of perfection. Embrace your uniqueness and acknowledge that you are worthy of love and acceptance just as you are.

Embracing self-compassion is an ongoing journey, one that requires patience and practice. It's a powerful tool that empowers us to embrace our authentic selves, nurture our well-being, and cultivate greater happiness and contentment in life.

When we continue on the path to a Happy New You, let us remember to be gentle and kind to ourselves. Let us release the burden of self-criticism and embrace our imperfections with open arms. May self-compassion be our guiding light, illuminating our journey with warmth, love, and acceptance. In the words of Kristin Neff, "You can't stop the waves, but you can learn to surf." Through self-compassion, we learn to navigate the waves of life with grace and resilience, riding them with self-acceptance and a compassionate heart.

> "I THINK IT'S IMPORTANT TO START THE DAY WITH A CLEAN SLATE, A CLEAR WORK ENVIRONMENT, AND A MADE BED."
>
> ALEXA VON TOBEL

CHAPTER 41
MAKE YOUR BED—A SMALL ACT WITH GREAT IMPACT

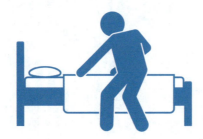

In the quest for a Happy New You, we often overlook the power of small actions that can set the tone for our day and pave the way for success. One such seemingly insignificant act is making your bed every morning, and its profound impact is beautifully depicted in William H. McRaven's book "Make Your Bed."

William McRaven, a retired U.S. Navy Admiral, shares powerful life lessons learned during his Navy SEAL training. The first lesson he imparts to his recruits is to make their beds each morning, even amidst the most grueling circumstances. You might wonder, "Why such emphasis on making a bed?" The answer lies in the ripple effect of this simple act.

Making your bed symbolizes starting the day with discipline, pride, and a sense of accomplishment. It creates an aura of order and control that can set a positive tone for the rest of your day. This small act can be the catalyst for bigger achievements and a step toward taking charge of your life.

As McRaven eloquently puts it, "If you make your bed every morning, you will have accomplished the first task of the day. It will give you a small sense of pride and encourage you to do another task and another."

It's the little things that add up over time, and making your bed is a testament to this truth. Success is built on a foundation of discipline and consistency, and forming the habit of making your bed can foster these qualities in your life.

Additionally, the act of making your bed extends its impact beyond your personal space. It sends a positive message to those around you, reinforcing the idea that you take pride in even the smallest aspects of your life. Your friends, family, and colleagues may witness your commitment to excellence, inspiring them to adopt similar habits.

Moreover, by starting your day with an accomplished task, you gain momentum to tackle more significant challenges throughout the day. Each accomplishment feeds into the next, creating a cycle of progress and self-assurance.

Just like McRaven's recruits, we may face storms and adversities in our lives. But amidst the chaos, making your bed can be an anchor of stability and control. It serves as a reminder that despite external challenges, you have the power to maintain order and positivity in your immediate surroundings.

The philosophy of making your bed also extends to other aspects of life. By mastering the discipline of small daily tasks, you build the resilience to face larger challenges with confidence. You become better equipped to deal with life's uncertainties and overcome obstacles in pursuit of your dreams.

So, let's take a lesson from Admiral McRaven and embrace the practice of making our beds each morning. As we smooth the sheets and fluff the pillows, let's remember that this simple act can lay the groundwork for an extraordinary day and a Happy New You.

In the grand tapestry of life, it's the seemingly insignificant threads that weave the most profound stories. And it all starts with making your bed.

"Start each day with a task completed. Find someone to help you through life. Respect everyone. Know that life is not fair, and that you will fail often. But if you take some risks, step up when times are toughest, face down the bullies, lift up the downtrodden, and never, ever give up – if you do these things, then the next generation and the generations that follow will live in a world far better than the one we have today." —Admiral William H. McRaven

> # MENTAL REHEARSAL IS JUST AS IMPORTANT AS PHYSICAL REHEARSAL.
>
> — BILLIE JEAN KING

CHAPTER 42
ACHIEVING GOLD WITH VISUALIZATION

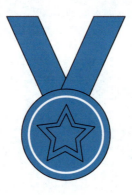

In this chapter, we dive into the extraordinary world of visualization and explore how Olympic athletes leverage its power to achieve the pinnacle of success: the Gold Medal. We will uncover the secrets behind their mental training and how you, too, can harness the power of visualization to accomplish your dreams.

Olympic athletes are masters of their craft, but their journey to victory begins long before they step onto the world stage. One of their most potent tools is the art of visualization. By creating detailed and vivid mental images of their performances, they tap into the immense power of their minds to shape their destinies.

Why Visualization Works

At first glance, visualization might seem like wishful thinking, but science has proven its efficacy. The brain doesn't distinguish between real and imagined experiences. When you visualize an action or outcome, the neural pathways in your brain fire in a way that's almost identical to the real experience.

Visualization plays a crucial role in learning, skill development, and performance improvement. By vividly imagining yourself accomplishing a task, your brain begins to build the neurological connections necessary to make that action a reality.

For Olympic athletes, visualization is like a secret weapon that enhances their physical training. It's a powerful mental rehearsal that primes them for success and sets them up to perform at their best under immense pressure.

The Power of Mental Rehearsal

An Olympic athlete envisions their performance, and they see every detail in their mind's eye. They visualize themselves executing every move with precision, feeling the sensations in their body, and hearing the cheers of the crowd. They focus on the desired outcome, whether it's crossing the finish line first or executing a flawless routine.

Michael Phelps, the most decorated Olympian in history, is a prime example of the power of visualization. Before each race, he would close his eyes and run a mental movie of the perfect swim, stroke by stroke, turn by turn. Phelps famously said, "I always visualize the race before I go. I've been doing it for so long that I can see the whole race."

The Neuroscience Behind Visualization

When athletes visualize themselves winning, their brains release neurotransmitters like dopamine and endorphins. These "feel-good" chemicals reinforce the neural connections associated with success, creating a positive feedback loop that fuels their confidence and motivation.

Visualization also activates the brain's reticular activating system (RAS), which filters information from the environment. By programming their RAS to focus on their goals, athletes become more aware of opportunities and resources that align with their vision, making it easier to achieve their objectives.

You Can Be an Olympic Visualization Champion, Too

You don't have to be an Olympic athlete to harness the power of visualization. Whether you're an entrepreneur, artist, student, or anyone with aspirations, visualization can be your key to unlocking untapped potential.

Clarify Your Vision

Clearly define your goals and dreams. Be specific and vividly imagine what success looks and feels like for you.

Engage Your Senses

When visualizing, engage all your senses. See the colors, hear the sounds, feel the sensations. Make the mental movie as real as possible.

Practice Regularly

Like physical training, mental rehearsal improves with practice. Dedicate time each day to visualize your success. Any time of the day will work, but I suggest doing it in the morning, so you start your day off right with how you want it to go.

Embrace Emotions

Feel the emotions associated with achieving your goals. Experience the joy, pride, and excitement as if you've already succeeded.

Visualize Challenges

Include challenges and obstacles in your visualizations. See yourself overcoming them with resilience and grace. By visualizing obstacles, you can build resilience and see obstacles as growth opportunities. Typically, we see obstacles as a negative, but by visualizing them you can start seeing how they can help move you toward your goals.

Create a Mental Playlist

Develop a playlist of positive affirmations and mantras that align with your vision. Repeat them daily to reinforce your belief in yourself.

Trust the Process

Stay patient and persistent. Trust that your visualization practice is aligning your subconscious mind with your goals.

Olympic athletes know that true victory starts with belief in their minds. They use visualization as a powerful tool to enhance their performance and achieve greatness. By adopting the Olympian's approach to visualization, you can unlock your full potential and set yourself on a course to achieve Gold in your life.

So, close your eyes and see yourself accomplishing your dreams. Embrace the emotions of success, and watch as your reality aligns with your visions. Visualization is your key to unlock the extraordinary life that awaits you.

> **THERE IS NO FAILURE EXCEPT IN NO LONGER TRYING.**
>
> — ELBERT HUBBARD

CHAPTER 43
EMBRACING FAILURE—THE COURAGE TO CONTINUE

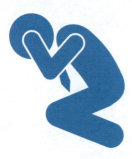

In our journey towards a Happy New You, one vital aspect that often gets overlooked is the power of embracing failure. It's essential to recognize that failure is not the end; instead, it is an opportunity to learn, grow, and evolve. As Winston Churchill wisely said, "Success is not final, failure is not fatal: it is the courage to continue that counts."

Throughout history, there have been numerous examples of individuals who faced countless rejections and setbacks but persevered to achieve greatness. One such remarkable story is that of Colonel Sanders, the founder of Kentucky Fried Chicken (KFC).

Colonel Sanders had a vision, a secret chicken recipe he believed would revolutionize the fast-food industry. He knocked on the doors of numerous restaurants, presenting his recipe and seeking an opportunity to partner with them. However, he was met with rejection, not once, not twice, but hundreds of times.

Most people would have given up after facing so much rejection, but not Colonel Sanders. He believed in his product, and he had the courage to continue. He traveled across the country, tirelessly promoting his recipe and looking for a partner who shared his vision. It wasn't an easy journey, but he refused to let failure define him.

Finally, after years of hard work and persistence, Colonel Sanders found the right partner, and KFC was born. Today, KFC is a global brand and one of the most successful fast-food chains in the world, all because one man had the courage to embrace failure and keep going.

The lesson here is that failure is not something to be feared or avoided. It is a stepping stone on the path to success. Each failure presents an opportunity to learn, adapt, and improve. It is through failure that we gain valuable insights and refine our approach.

When you encounter failure, don't let it discourage you. Instead, view it as an essential part of the learning process. Take the time to reflect on what went wrong, identify areas for improvement, and use that knowledge to make better decisions in the future.

Embracing failure also means letting go of the fear of judgment and the pressure to be perfect. It's okay to make mistakes; it's part of being human. What matters is how we respond to those mistakes and setbacks. We can choose to see them as opportunities for growth or as reasons to give up.

When you find yourself facing failure, remember the story of Colonel Sanders and countless other individuals who didn't let rejection define them. They chose to keep going, to learn from their mistakes, and to continue striving for their goals.

In your own life, whether it's in your personal or professional endeavors, embrace failure as a natural part of the journey toward success. Cultivate resilience, perseverance, and the courage to keep moving forward.

As you continue pursuing a Happy New You, remember that failure is not the end of the road; it's just a detour. With every setback, you gain valuable experience and become better equipped to achieve your dreams. So, have the courage to continue, and let failure be a stepping stone to your ultimate success.

> # FEAR IS ONLY AS DEEP AS THE MIND ALLOWS.
>
> JAPANESE PROVERB

CHAPTER 44
TRANSFORMING FEAR INTO POWER— BREAKING THROUGH LIMITING BELIEFS

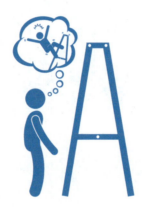

Fear. It's a powerful emotion that can hold us back from reaching our true potential and living a life of fulfillment. But what if I told you that fear is nothing more than False Evidence Appearing Real? That's right—fear is often just an illusion, a product of our imagination that prevents us from taking the actions needed to achieve greatness.

In this chapter, we are going to explore the art of transforming fear into power. We'll discover how to break through the walls of limiting beliefs and unleash our true potential. The journey won't be easy, but it will be worth it.

Let me share with you a real-life story of someone who did just that. At a Tony Robbins event, I had the privilege of meeting a remarkable woman named Rhonda. She found herself facing the daunting challenge of breaking a board with her bare hand. She was terrified, ready to run away and hide. But she decided to stay and face her fear head-on.

As Rhonda stood in front of that board, heart pounding, palms sweaty, and doubts creeping in, she realized that breaking the board wasn't just about physical strength. It was a metaphor for breaking through her own self-doubt and limiting beliefs. With a surge of courage, she took a deep breath and summoned all the power within her.

And in that moment, something incredible happened. Rhonda broke through the board, shattering not only the wood but also the barriers of fear that held her back for so long. It was a transformative experience that forever changed her life.

You see, breaking through fear isn't about physical feats; it's about the mindset shift that occurs when we confront our fears head-on. It's about realizing that fear is just an illusion—a story we tell ourselves. And, like any story, we have the power to rewrite it.

Tony Robbins once said, "It is in your moments of decision that your destiny is shaped." What he meant by this profound statement is that the choices we make, especially in the face of fear, have the power to shape our lives. Each decision to confront fear and push through it propels us toward our destiny, creating a life filled with purpose and passion.

So, how can you transform fear into power in your own life? Start by acknowledging your fears and recognizing them for what they are—False Evidence Appearing Real. Embrace and accept them. Next, challenge those fears with evidence of your capabilities and past successes. Remind yourself of the times you conquered fear and achieved greatness. And remember to breathe. Deep breathing taps into the calming part of her nervous system, allowing us to have a better perspective.

Surround yourself with a support system that believes in you and encourages you to step outside your comfort zone. Seek guidance from mentors and coaches who have overcome their own fears and can show you the way.

Most importantly, be patient and compassionate with yourself. Breaking through fear is a process, and it's okay to take small steps. Celebrate every victory, no matter how small, and use them as stepping stones towards greater accomplishments.

As you embark on this journey of transforming fear into power, remember Rhonda's board break and the courage she summoned to face her fears. Embrace the challenge, break through the barriers, and transform fear into power—the power to live your Happy New You life to the fullest, with a destiny shaped by the decisions you make.

> "SHOW ME A SUCCESSFUL INDIVIDUAL, AND I'LL SHOW YOU SOMEONE WHO HAD REAL POSITIVE INFLUENCES IN HIS OR HER LIFE. I DON'T CARE WHAT YOU DO FOR A LIVING- IF YOU DO IT WELL, I AM SURE THERE WAS SOMEONE CHEERING YOU ON OR SHOWING YOU THE WAY. A MENTOR.
>
> — DENZEL WASHINGTON"

CHAPTER 45

THE POWER OF MENTORSHIP AND CONTINUOUS LEARNING

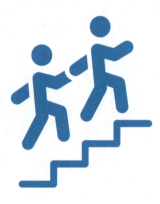

In our journey towards a Happy New You, one of the most transformative elements is the power of mentorship and continuous learning. Throughout life, we have the opportunity to be both a mentee and a mentor, each role offering valuable insights and wisdom.

I want to share with you the profound impact my mentor, Pavel Tsatsouline, has had on my life. Pavel is a renowned strength and conditioning coach, known for his expertise in kettlebell training and physical performance. His teachings have not only shaped my physical capabilities but have also instilled valuable lessons that extend far beyond the gym.

One of the fundamental principles Pavel emphasized is the importance of deliberate practice. It's not just about mindlessly going through the motions but actively focusing on every aspect of your practice to achieve mastery. Being mindful, thinking about what you are doing and not just going through the motions. This concept applies not only to physical training but also to all aspects of life.

Through Pavel's guidance, I learned the value of setting clear goals and breaking them down into manageable steps. This approach empowered me to make progress, even in the face of challenging obstacles. And as I achieved those milestones, my self confidence soared, reinforcing the belief that anything is possible with the right mindset and dedication. He helped take me from a broken body, ready to give up my career, to a strong, capable body that is able to work without issues.

Mentorship extends beyond one-on-one relationships. There is an abundance of knowledge and wisdom to be gained from books, courses, and seminars. Continuous learning is the fuel that drives personal growth and development. By immersing ourselves in new perspectives and ideas, we expand our horizons and tap into our true potential.

Just as Pavel's mentorship has been pivotal in my life, I encourage you to seek out mentors and sources of knowledge that resonate with your passions and goals. Surround yourself with individuals who inspire and challenge you to become the best version of yourself.

Mentorship is a two-way street, and as we gain insights from our mentors, we also have the opportunity to give back and mentor others. Sharing our experiences and wisdom creates a ripple effect of positive change, uplifting not only ourselves but those we touch along the way.

Continuous learning is an ongoing journey, and it's essential to approach it with an open mind and a thirst for knowledge. Embrace new experiences, seek out different perspectives, and be willing to explore unfamiliar territories. Remember that learning is not confined to formal education; it can be found in everyday interactions and experiences.

In our rapidly changing world, continuous learning is more critical than ever. It equips us with the adaptability and resilience needed to thrive amidst uncertainty and challenges. Embrace the growth mindset, seeing every setback as an opportunity to learn and improve.

As we integrate mentorship and continuous learning into our lives, we tap into an infinite reservoir of potential. By seeking guidance, sharing our wisdom, and immersing ourselves in the constant pursuit of knowledge, we unlock the power to transform our lives and create a Happy New You, filled with purpose, fulfillment, and growth.

The concept of becoming the equal of the five people you spend the most time with is a powerful one. It suggests that our environment and the people we surround ourselves with significantly shape our beliefs, attitudes, and behaviors.

Think about the five people you spend the most time with. Are they positive, driven individuals who inspire and challenge you to grow? Or do they bring negativity and drag you down? It's essential to be conscious of the company we keep and how it affects our mindset and actions. It does matter.

When we surround ourselves with successful, ambitious, and supportive individuals, we absorb their energy and enthusiasm. They motivate us to aim higher, embrace challenges, and strive for excellence. On the other hand, negative influences can drain our energy, create self-doubt, and hinder our progress.

To foster personal growth, seek out relationships with people who uplift and encourage you. Be open to making new connections and joining communities aligned with your goals and interests. Attend seminars, workshops, or networking events to meet like-minded individuals on similar paths.

Additionally, immerse yourself in learning from mentors and role models who have achieved what you aspire to accomplish. Learn from their experiences, setbacks, and successes, and let their wisdom guide your own journey.

Remember that mentorship and personal development go hand in hand. As you invest in continuous learning, you cultivate your ability to be a mentor to others. Share your insights, experiences, and knowledge with those around you, and contribute to their growth and transformation.

By becoming intentional about the company we keep, we elevate our standards and expectations for ourselves. We learn from others' achievements and setbacks, drawing inspiration to overcome our challenges and embrace opportunities.

As you journey towards a Happy New You, remember that your growth and transformation are influenced by your commitment to mentorship and continuous learning. Embrace the power of surrounding yourself with positive, driven individuals, and let their support propel you towards your dreams and aspirations. In the process, you become not only the sum of your experiences but also the average of the five people you choose to walk this path with.

> # SOMEDAY IS NOT A DAY OF THE WEEK.
>
> ---
> JANET DAILEY

CHAPTER 46
OVERCOMING PROCRASTINATION AND TAKING ACTION WITH THE 5 SECOND RULE

In this chapter, we will explore a powerful tool to conquer procrastination and unleash your potential—Mel Robbins' "The 5 Second Rule." Procrastination is a common struggle that many people face, but it doesn't have to hold you back any longer. Let's dive into the depths of this transformative concept and learn how to break free from self-sabotage.

Mel Robbins, a renowned motivational speaker and author, introduced the world to "The 5 Second Rule" as a game-changing technique to take control of your thoughts and actions. It's a simple but incredibly effective method to beat procrastination and hesitation, and it's designed to help you take immediate action towards your goals and dreams.

The concept is quite straightforward—when you find yourself hesitating or feeling overwhelmed, count down from 5 to 1, and then immediately take action. The countdown serves as a trigger to interrupt any negative thought patterns and propel you into action before self-doubt and fear can take over.

You see, procrastination often stems from fear of failure or a lack of confidence in our abilities. We hesitate, we overthink, and we self-sabotage. But remember, you are not a failure for procrastinating; it's a common human behavior. The key is to recognize it and take steps to change it.

"The 5 Second Rule" empowers you to bypass the mental barriers that hold you back and tap into your potential. It's a tool that can be used in various aspects of life, from tackling daunting tasks at work to making healthier lifestyle choices.

So how does it work? Let's break it down.

Recognize the Hesitation

Pay attention to the moments when you start to hesitate or doubt yourself. It could be when you're about to make a phone call, start a project, or take a step toward your dreams. As soon as you say, "I should go exercise, eat something good, do my homework, write that book…." Look for what comes next. If your brain says I don't need to, I don't want to, I can't, just know it is looking for a safe way out, and you can't listen to it. You have five seconds, or you are going to give in.

Count Down from 5

As soon as you notice that hesitation, start counting down from 5 to 1—5, 4, 3, 2, 1. When you reach "1," push yourself to take immediate action. Make the phone call, open your laptop, or take that first step.

By following this simple rule, you can interrupt the negative thought patterns and shift your focus towards action. You'll be amazed at how powerful this technique can be in breaking the cycle of procrastination. The book "The 5 Second Rule" offers several additional strategies to help you apply this principle to various aspects of your life.

Morning Ritual

Use the 5 Second Rule to jump-start your day with a positive and productive mindset. When your alarm goes off in the morning, count down from 5 and get out of bed immediately. This simple action sets the tone for the rest of your day and helps you avoid hitting the snooze button and falling into a cycle of sluggishness.

Overcoming Fear and Anxiety

The 5 Second Rule can be particularly effective in moments of fear and anxiety. Whether you're about to give a presentation, approach someone new, or face a challenging situation, counting down from 5 can help you gather the courage to take the necessary action and overcome your fears.

Navigating Procrastination

The book offers additional insights on how to navigate procrastination and create lasting behavior changes. Mel Robbins delves into the science behind the rule and provides practical advice on how to make it a permanent part of your life.

"The 5 Second Rule" is a valuable tool that empowers you to break free from self-sabotage and take decisive action toward your dreams. By using this simple countdown technique, you can rewire your brain and create positive habits that lead to lasting success.

Make "The 5 Second Rule" a part of your daily life and empower yourself to take decisive action. You have the strength within you to break free from procrastination, conquer your doubts, and achieve the life you desire. Embrace the power of taking action and step into your greatness. Your Happy New You awaits!

> TO LOSE PATIENCE IS TO LOSE THE BATTLE.
>
> — MAHATMA GANDHI

CHAPTER 47
CULTIVATING PATIENCE— TRUSTING THE PROCESS OF GROWTH

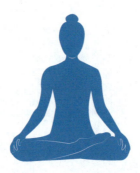

In the pursuit of your Happy New You, one of the most valuable virtues to embrace is patience. Cultivating patience allows you to navigate life's challenges with grace, maintain a positive mindset, and trust in the natural process of growth and transformation. Here are ten tried and proven tips to help you cultivate patience in your life.

Practice Mindfulness

Bring awareness to your thoughts and emotions without judgment. Mindfulness helps you observe impatience as it arises and choose a more patient response. Deep breathing with mindfulness helps you to slow down, giving you the ability to be patient.

Embrace Acceptance

Recognize that some things are beyond your control. Embracing acceptance allows you to let go of the need for immediate outcomes and trust in divine timing.

Set Realistic Expectations

Be realistic about the time it takes to achieve your goals. Avoid setting rigid deadlines and acknowledge that success is a journey, not an instant destination. Nothing changes in an instant, and the sooner we realize it the calmer we can be in our journey. You are not going to lose 50 pounds in one month, and you are not going to make a million dollars within the next 6 weeks.

Breathe and Center Yourself

When faced with moments of impatience, take a deep breath and center yourself. This simple act can bring a sense of calm and clarity.

Practice Gratitude

Focus on the blessings and progress you've already made. Most of us focus on what still needs to be done, but if we shift our thinking to how far we have gotten, we can have patience with our next steps. Gratitude shifts your perspective and helps you recognize the beauty in each step of your journey.

Seek Perspective

Step back from challenging situations and consider the bigger picture. Seeking perspective reminds you that setbacks are temporary and part of the learning process.

Practice Delayed Gratification

Train yourself to delay immediate rewards for greater long-term benefits. This skill enhances your ability to be patient with the process. I grew up in an era where we lived in delayed gratification. We didn't have credit cards, so we had to save for what we wanted. When we ordered things out of a catalogue it would take 8 weeks to show up. It is too easy to get "things" these days and there is no delaying anything. Ask yourself, "Do I really need this?" before hitting buy. Practicing delayed gratification helps you get closer to your goals.

Cultivate Compassion

Show compassion to yourself and others. Recognize that everyone has their own journey, and growth takes time and effort.

Celebrate Progress

Acknowledge and celebrate even the smallest victories. Celebrating progress reinforces patience and fuels your motivation to keep going.

Engage in Self-Care

Take care of your physical and emotional well-being. Engaging in self-care helps you build resilience, making it easier to remain patient during challenging times.

By incorporating these ten tips into your daily life, you can cultivate the art of patience and trust in the process of growth. Remember that just like a flower needs time to blossom, your personal development also requires nurturing and time to reach its full potential.

Be gentle with yourself as you navigate the journey of patience. It's not about being perfect; it's about progress. Embrace the process, trust in your abilities, and know that every step forward, no matter how small, is a step towards your Happy New You. As you practice patience, you'll find peace, joy, and fulfillment, and your life will flourish in ways you never imagined.

So, take a deep breath, embrace the present moment, and trust in the unfolding of your beautiful journey. Cultivate patience as a powerful tool on your path to creating the life you truly desire.

> **CHANGE IS HARD AT FIRST, MESSY IN THE MIDDLE, AND GORGEOUS AT THE END.**
>
> ROBIN SHARMA

CHAPTER 48

EMBRACING CHANGE— THRIVING IN TIMES OF TRANSITION

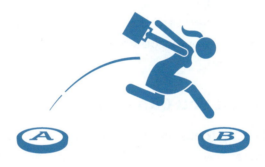

In the midst of a rapidly changing world, it's natural to feel uncertain and uneasy about the future. The truth is, that change is an inevitable part of life, and it presents us with both challenges and opportunities. As we navigate through these uncharted waters, let's remember the quote from Robert H. Schuller, "Tough times never last, but tough people do." Change can be unsettling, but it also holds the potential for growth, resilience, and progress.

Throughout history, some of the greatest advancements and breakthroughs have emerged from times of profound change. The world faced the devastating impact of the Great Depression, yet it laid the foundation for economic reforms and social progress that improved the lives of many. Similarly, the aftermath of World War II led to an era of global cooperation and prosperity.

Embracing change doesn't mean dismissing the difficulties it may bring. Instead, it involves acknowledging the challenges while maintaining a positive and adaptable mindset. We must embrace the unknown. Here are some empowering insights to help you thrive in times of transition.

The Courage to Explore

Instead of fearing the unknown, approach it with curiosity and openness. Embracing the unfamiliar can lead to discoveries and opportunities you never thought possible. Just like explorers, venturing into uncharted territories gives you the courage to step into the unknown and embrace change as a catalyst for personal growth and evolution.

Focus on What You Can Control

In times of change, focus on the aspects of your life that you can control. Let go of the rest, and channel your energy into actions that can bring positive results. Life is unpredictable, but your adaptability and resourcefulness can be unwavering. By accepting that change is a constant, you'll find the strength to overcome challenges and navigate through transitions with resilience.

Stay Committed to Your Goals

While circumstances may change, your goals and values can remain constant. Stay committed to your vision and be flexible in finding new paths to achieve it. Like a sailor steering through stormy seas, keep your purpose as your guiding North Star. Align your actions with your long-term goals and let them be your anchor during times of uncertainty.

Seek Support

During challenging times, it's essential to lean on your support system. Connect with friends, family, or mentors who can provide guidance and encouragement. The beauty of human connection lies in the ability to uplift and inspire one another. Seek comfort in the embrace of your support network and find solace in the fact that you are not alone on this journey.

Practice Resilience

Cultivate resilience by adapting to new situations and bouncing back from setbacks. Resilience is the key to navigating change with grace and strength. Like a tree bending in the face of a storm, your ability to bend without breaking will determine your growth and survival. Embrace change as an opportunity to discover your inner strength and resilience.

Learn from the Past

History shows us that change is a catalyst for growth. Look back at how humanity has overcome adversities in the past and draw inspiration from those stories. The wisdom of the past can guide your steps in the present and shape your decisions for the future. Learn from the experiences of those who came before you and use their wisdom as a beacon of hope. Also, remember that the past doesn't equal the future. Use the past to learn what or what not to do as you go forward.

See Change as an Opportunity

Instead of viewing change as a threat, see it as an opportunity for personal and collective growth. Change can pave the way for innovation and progress. Just like the butterfly emerging from its cocoon, change can lead to the blossoming of new talents, ideas, and possibilities. Embrace the winds of change and let them carry you to new heights.

Maintain a Positive Mindset

Amidst uncertainty, a positive mindset can be a guiding light. Focus on the possibilities that lie ahead and maintain an optimistic outlook. By cultivating a positive attitude, you'll be better equipped to find solutions and discover hidden opportunities, even in the face of adversity. Saying "I can" will help propel you forward.

Take Care of Yourself

During times of change, self-care is crucial. Prioritize your physical and emotional well-being to stay strong and adaptable. Like a gardener nurturing a young plant, take care of yourself so you can weather the storms and bloom in the sunlight. Nurture your body, mind, and soul to maintain a balanced foundation for growth and transformation.

Embrace Lifelong Learning

Embrace change as an opportunity for continuous learning and personal development. Stay curious, and be open to acquiring new skills and knowledge. Life is a never-ending journey of growth and learning, and every change presents a chance to evolve into a better version of yourself.

As you embrace change and navigate times of transition, remember that you have the power to shape your own destiny. Embrace change as an invitation to evolve, adapt, and grow. The world may be in flux, but you have the inner strength and resilience to thrive in the face of uncertainty.

The journey of embracing change is an opportunity to uncover your untapped potential and uncover the greatness within you. Just as the phoenix rises from the ashes, you, too, can emerge stronger and wiser from the challenges you encounter.

Now, let's take a moment to acknowledge that some of the insights we've shared in this chapter might sound familiar to you. That's because, in previous chapters, we discussed powerful tools and concepts that apply just as strongly to navigating change as they do to other aspects of your life.

In the pursuit of your Happy New You, remember the importance of cultivating patience, embracing gratitude, visualizing your success, and practicing the art of self-compassion. These powerful habits can bolster your resilience and help you thrive in the face of change.

So, let's reinforce these foundational habits as you embrace the winds of change. When the tides of life shift, remember to draw from your reservoir of inner strength and adaptability. Together, let's navigate the waves of change and embrace the adventure of a lifetime! Tough times may come, but you possess the tenacity, courage, and resilience to overcome any storm that comes your way. Embrace the winds of change and let them carry you towards the life of purpose, fulfillment, and joy that awaits you.

> **EMPATHY IS THE MEDICINE THE WORLD NEEDS.**
>
> — JUDITH ORLOFF, MD

CHAPTER 49
THE POWER OF EMPATHY— CONNECTING WITH OTHERS' HEARTS

In a world filled with chaos and uncertainty, the value of empathy has never been more evident. Empathy is the ability to understand and share the feelings of others, and it serves as a powerful bridge that connects us on a deeper, more compassionate level. As we navigate the challenges of today's world, let us recognize the profound impact that empathy can have on our lives and the lives of those around us.

Think about the last time you encountered someone driving recklessly on the freeway, cutting in and out of traffic without any regard for others. Our initial response might be frustration or anger, as we witness this dangerous behavior affecting everyone around us. But what if, for a moment, we chose empathy? What if we considered that there might be more to the story?

Perhaps the person speeding down the freeway just received a distressing phone call that their wife has been rushed to the emergency room. Or maybe they are racing to be with a loved one who is in crisis and needs their immediate support. By choosing empathy, we allow ourselves to step into their shoes and understand that their actions might be driven by fear, urgency, or desperation.

Empathy isn't just about being understanding; it's about recognizing our shared humanity. It's about acknowledging that every person we encounter is experiencing their own struggles, triumphs, and challenges. When we open our hearts to empathy, we create a ripple effect of kindness and compassion that can uplift not only our own lives but the lives of others as well.

Here are some profound ways in which empathy can transform our lives.

Cultivating Emotional Resilience

By practicing empathy, we become emotionally resilient. When we understand that everyone is fighting their own battles, it helps us put our challenges into perspective and approach them with a calmer, more composed mindset. Empathy allows us to process emotions more clearly, leading to better decision-making and problem-solving.

Strengthening Relationships

Empathy forms the foundation of meaningful relationships. When we listen, truly listen, to others and seek to understand their feelings, we build trust and intimacy. Our connections deepen, and we create an environment of support and compassion.

Empathy fosters an atmosphere of love and respect, strengthening the bonds we share with friends, family, and colleagues.

Reducing Conflict and Misunderstandings

Misunderstandings and conflicts often arise from a lack of empathy. When we dismiss or invalidate others' emotions, it can lead to tension and discord. On the other hand, empathy promotes open communication and allows us to find common ground. By seeking to understand one another, we create a space for dialogue and compromise.

Encouraging Acts of Kindness

Empathy inspires acts of kindness and generosity. When we recognize the struggles of others, we are more inclined to extend a helping hand. From simple gestures of kindness to more significant acts of service, empathy compels us to make a positive difference in the lives of those around us.

Boosting Emotional Intelligence

Empathy is a cornerstone of emotional intelligence. When we understand and manage our emotions, we become more attuned to the feelings of others. This heightened emotional intelligence enables us to navigate social situations with grace and empathy, fostering deeper connections and more meaningful interactions.

Nurturing Self-Compassion

Practicing empathy towards others helps us develop self-compassion as well. When we embrace our own imperfections and struggles, we are more forgiving and understanding of ourselves. Empathy reminds us that we are all on a journey of growth and self-discovery, and it's okay to be imperfect.

Empowering Positive Change

Empathy fuels our desire for positive change. When we empathize with the suffering and injustices in the world, we are motivated to take action. Empathy can drive us to stand up for what is right, advocate for those in need, and contribute to the betterment of society.

As we cultivate empathy, we become beacons of light in a world that can sometimes feel dark and uncertain. Our capacity to empathize allows us to create a supportive and compassionate community where everyone feels seen, heard, and valued.

In times of distress or conflict, let empathy be your guiding light. When faced with challenging situations, pause for a moment and ask yourself, "How would I feel if I were in their shoes?" This simple question can transform your perspective and open your heart to a deeper understanding of others.

The journey of empathy begins with small acts of kindness and understanding. Start by actively listening to others without judgment, and seek to understand their experiences and emotions. Be present with those around you, and offer a compassionate ear when someone needs to talk.

Remember that empathy is not about fixing someone's problems or taking on their burdens. It's about holding space for others and validating their emotions. Sometimes, all a person needs is to be heard and understood.

In the pursuit of your Happy New You, let empathy guide your interactions and decisions. Practice it not only towards others but also towards yourself. By nurturing empathy, you'll create a profound impact on your own well-being and the well-being of the world around you.

As we journey through the changing landscape of the world, let empathy be the guiding force that connects our hearts and uplifts our spirits. Together, let's create a more compassionate and understanding world, one act of empathy at a time.

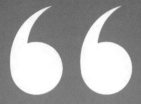

BE NOT AFRAID OF GOING SLOWLY, BE AFRAID ONLY OF STANDING STILL.

CHINESE PROVERB

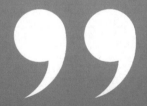

CHAPTER 50
TRACK YOUR PROGRESS—CELEBRATING YOUR WINS AND SUSTAINING YOUR HAPPY NEW YOU JOURNEY

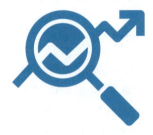

Congratulations! You've embarked on a transformative journey with "Happy New You" that has ignited the flames of positive change in your life. As you reach this milestone, let us take a moment to reflect on the progress you've made and the remarkable transformation that awaits you.

"Happy New You" has served as your launching pad, propelling you into a year of growth, self-discovery, and empowerment. But it doesn't end here; it's merely the beginning of a lifelong journey towards creating a Happy New Year, year after year, filled with joy, fulfillment, and success.

One of the most potent tools in your arsenal for sustaining this progress is tracking your journey. By monitoring your growth, celebrating your wins, and learning from challenges, you're creating a roadmap to your Happy New Year success. So, let's delve into the power of tracking your progress and how it can shape the trajectory of your life.

Celebrate Your Wins

Take a moment to celebrate every milestone, big or small, that you've achieved on this journey. Whether it's completing a self-improvement challenge, overcoming a fear, or achieving a goal, celebrate yourself for the dedication and effort you've put in. Celebrating your wins not only boosts your confidence and self-esteem but also serves as a reminder of your progress and motivates you to keep moving forward.

Learn from Challenges

As you track your progress, you'll inevitably encounter challenges along the way. Embrace these challenges as opportunities for growth and learning. Reflect on the lessons you've gained from facing obstacles, and remember that every setback is a stepping stone to greater resilience and wisdom. Write down the challenges and what good might come from them, how they might change your journey for the better, or how you might pivot in a different direction that you didn't see possible.

Set New Goals

Tracking your progress enables you to assess where you are and where you want to go. As you celebrate your wins and overcome challenges, consider setting new goals for yourself. These goals can be an extension of the ones you've already achieved or entirely new aspirations that align with your evolving vision of a Happy New Year.

Stay Committed to Self-Improvement

The journey to a Happy New You is an ongoing commitment to self-improvement. As you track your progress, you'll witness the incredible impact of consistent efforts over time. Embrace the mindset of continuous growth and be open to new opportunities for learning and personal development.

Create Lasting Habits

Tracking your progress reinforces positive habits that you've cultivated throughout the year. These habits are the foundation of your success, and by consistently tracking your efforts, you solidify them as a part of your lifestyle. Remember, the key to lasting change lies in the daily habits you embrace.

Be Kind to Yourself

In the pursuit of progress, be kind and compassionate to yourself. Acknowledge that growth is a journey with ups and downs. No progress is in a straight line, even if someone else's Facebook shows that. If you encounter moments of stagnation or setbacks, remind yourself that it's all part of the process. Your self-compassion and determination will help you stay on track and continue your journey towards a Happy New You.

Embrace the Power of Gratitude

In your tracking journey, don't forget to cultivate gratitude for the abundance in your life. Gratitude has a profound effect on your overall well-being and outlook on life. By acknowledging the blessings and opportunities that come your way, you invite more positivity and happiness into your daily existence.

As you continue to track your progress, remember that this journey is not about perfection; it's about growth, resilience, and embracing the beauty of the process. Your Happy New Year is a mosaic of moments, experiences, and personal triumphs that shape your life in meaningful ways.

So, let "Happy New You" be the catalyst that fuels your ongoing journey towards creating a Happy New Year for years to come. With each passing year, you'll have a wealth of accomplishments, insights, and memories to look back upon with gratitude and pride.

As you embark on this lifelong journey, know that you have the power to shape your destiny and craft a life filled with joy, purpose, and fulfillment. By tracking your progress and celebrating every step forward, you're sowing the seeds of a Happy New You that will blossom into a Happy New Year, year after year.

So, let's raise a toast to the incredible progress you've made and the limitless possibilities that lie ahead. Here's to a life of endless growth, joy, and success. Cheers to your Happy New You!

> **THE MOMENT YOU TAKE RESPONSIBILITY FOR EVERYTHING IN YOUR LIFE IS THE MOMENT YOU CAN CHANGE ANYTHING IN YOUR LIFE.**
>
> — HAL ELROD

CHAPTER 51
THE POWER OF OWNERSHIP— EMBRACE YOUR DESTINY WITH 100% RESPONSIBILITY

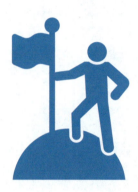

Congratulations on reaching Chapter 51! By embarking on this journey of self-discovery and empowerment, you've taken a significant step towards creating the life you desire. As you delve deeper into the essence of Happy New You, it's time to embrace a transformative principle that can alter the course of your life forever —taking 100% responsibility for your life. Take responsibility for all of it; the good, the bad, and the ugly. We are all human and are not perfect. Blaming other people for our issues doesn't help us but hinders us, it keeps us stuck in a life we do not want.

Life is a masterpiece woven with threads of choices, actions, and beliefs. It's easy to get caught up in the narrative of blaming circumstances, external forces, or other people for our challenges and setbacks. But here's a truth you need to hear loud and clear: No one is coming to rescue you. It is up to you to shape your destiny.

"The buck stops here." These simple but powerful words by President Harry S. Truman encapsulate the essence of taking ownership of your life. Embracing 100% responsibility means acknowledging that you are the architect of your reality, and every decision, big or small, shapes the course of your life.

Celebrate Your Journey

As you stand here in Chapter 51, take a moment to celebrate yourself. Celebrate the fact that you've come this far by embracing the wisdom and insights shared in "Happy New You." You've chosen to embark on a path of growth, self-improvement, and empowerment. Your dedication and willingness to change deserve applause.

The Gift of Ownership

One of the greatest gifts you can ever give yourself is taking ownership of your life. When you fully embrace this principle, you reclaim the power that might have been scattered across external circumstances and people. By accepting responsibility for your life, you become the driver of your journey, steering it towards the destination of your dreams. Not owing your life puts you in victim mode, which never allows for change.

The Mirror of Self-Reflection

Look in the mirror and recognize the person staring back at you as the captain of your ship. Yes, life can throw storms your way, but how you navigate through them lies within your control. By taking 100% responsibility, you step into your own strength and resilience.

Owning Your Setbacks

As you claim responsibility for your life, it's essential to recognize that setbacks and challenges are a part of the human experience. However, how you respond to them determines your growth and progress. Instead of placing blame elsewhere, embrace setbacks as opportunities for learning and growth. Every obstacle is a chance to refine your character and sharpen your skills.

Empowering Mindset Shifts

Taking ownership involves fostering a mindset that empowers you to be the architect of your reality. Here are some empowering shifts to incorporate into your life.

Focus on What You Can Control

Direct your energy towards things you can influence rather than dwelling on factors beyond your reach.

Embrace Accountability

Hold yourself accountable for your actions, choices, and outcomes. When you do so, you gain the power to direct your life's trajectory.

Let Go of Victimhood

Shed the cloak of victimhood and step into the role of a creator. By releasing the victim mindset, you open the door to unlimited possibilities. Staying in a victim mentality worsens our guilt and shame and can cause depression and anxiety.

My niece was bullied in school, and she didn't feel safe. For several years, she was very depressed and could hardly get out of bed. One day, she decided to make a change. She started getting up 15 minutes early before school and exercised her body with weights. She did this five days out of the week and took the weekends off. She now feels more confident and stronger. She took a bad situation and empowered herself to make a change. She chose not to be a victim but a victor, completely changing the path of her life.

Cultivate Resilience

Life may throw curveballs, but your ability to bounce back and adapt is a testament to your strength.

Learn from Mistakes

Embrace mistakes as opportunities for growth and learning. View them as stepping stones towards success.

The Ripple Effect of Ownership

By taking 100% responsibility for your life, you inspire others to do the same. Your actions and mindset create a ripple effect, positively impacting the lives of those around you. As you embody this principle, you become a beacon of empowerment and possibility.

Creating Your Happy New Year

With ownership as your guiding principle, you're equipped to design a Happy New Year that transcends any external circumstances. You're in control of the narrative, and you have the power to shape your reality in alignment with your dreams and aspirations.

So, as you embrace 100% responsibility, remember that you have the power to transform your life. Celebrate your journey, embrace setbacks, and take charge of your destiny. By doing so, you unleash the limitless potential within you and craft a life that truly reflects your heart's desires.

In the words of Mel Robbins, "You need to hear this loud and clear: No one is coming. It is up to you." With the power of ownership in your hands, you hold the key to a Happy New Year and a Happy New You—now and for all the years to come.

> **TRANSFORMATION ISN'T A FUTURE EVENT. IT'S A PRESENT-DAY ACTIVITY.**
>
> — JILLIAN MICHAELS

CHAPTER 52
CELEBRATING YOUR HAPPY NEW YOU—REFLECTING ON A YEAR OF GROWTH AND TRANSFORMATION

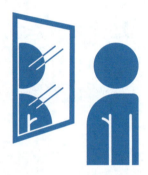

Congratulations on reaching the final chapter of "Happy New You—52 Habits to Creating the Life You Want!" As you stand at this milestone, take a moment to pat yourself on the back. You've journeyed through 52 weeks of self-discovery, empowerment, and transformation, and it's time to celebrate the incredible progress you've made.

Embrace Your Transformation

Over the course of this book (and year), you've dug deep into the essence of Happy New You, incorporating powerful habits and mindset shifts into your daily life. You've cultivated gratitude, embraced change, and taken 100% responsibility for your destiny.

You've nurtured a growth mindset, practiced self-compassion, and learned to set empowering goals. Each chapter has been a stepping stone towards creating the life you desire.

Share Your Story

Your journey to a Happy New You is not just about you; it's a powerful inspiration for others. As you celebrate your transformation, consider sharing your experiences, insights, and progress with the world. Post your stories and pictures on social media platforms like Facebook, Instagram, and Twitter, using the hashtags #HappyNewYou and #HappyNewYouTransformation.

By sharing your journey, you become a beacon of hope and motivation for those who may be seeking a positive change in their lives. Your story has the potential to touch lives, ignite sparks of inspiration, and create a ripple effect of transformation in the lives of others.

Spreading the Message of Happy New You

Your journey doesn't end with this book; it's a continuous cycle of growth and evolution. As you celebrate your achievements, consider sharing "Happy New You" with friends, family, and colleagues. The principles and insights you've gained can serve as a guiding light for others seeking positive change in their lives.

Epilogue: The Journey of Invisible Growth

In the heart of our transformative voyage through "Happy New You!" I shared with you countless tools, stories, and strategies aimed at catalyzing a profound inner metamorphosis. As we draw this journey to a close, I want to leave you with a tale that beautifully encapsulates the essence of our shared experience: the story of the Chinese bamboo.

Imagine planting a bamboo seed in your backyard. You care for it diligently, providing it with water, shielding it from the harsh sun, and ensuring it's free from pests. Days turn into weeks, weeks morph into months, and before you know it, years have passed. Yet, for four long years, despite your unwavering care, there's no visible sign of life above the soil. To an outsider, it may seem as though your efforts have been in vain. Then, in the fifth year, a miracle unfolds. From that seemingly dormant soil, a shoot springs forth, surging upwards at an astonishing rate, reaching almost 80 feet within weeks!

This astonishing growth isn't a result of the efforts of the fifth year alone but of the four preceding years during which the bamboo was silently, tenaciously laying a vast network of roots. These roots, invisible to the eye, are what prepared the bamboo for its rapid ascent when the time was right.

Why, you might ask, am I telling you about the bamboo in the closing chapter of "Happy New You!" The answer is simple yet profound: You, my dear friends, are that bamboo.

Throughout our journey, we delved deep into the realms of growth, self-awareness, self-actualization, and change. Much like nurturing the bamboo, there have been times when you've put in the work, yet felt like nothing was changing. This is natural, and it's vital to understand that much of personal development operates beneath the surface. Every insight you've gained, every habit you've tried to inculcate, and every reflection you've indulged in, is akin to the bamboo's roots spreading out beneath the ground. You might not see the changes instantly, but they are taking shape, building a robust foundation for the magnificent growth that lies ahead.

Change, especially the kind that lasts, is often silent and incremental. You're on a path of growth and evolution, and while some transformations might be evident, many will be subtle, working their magic in the background, preparing you for the leaps and bounds that await. And just like the bamboo, when the time is right, you'll find yourself rising, reaching heights you'd never imagined, and looking back with awe at the journey that got you there.

"Happy New You!" is not just a book; it's a philosophy, a way of life. The journey of self-improvement is continuous, and even after turning the final page, I urge you to keep the spirit of the book alive. Revisit the chapters from time to time. Just as a gardener tends to a bamboo plant long before its growth is visible, you, too, must continuously nurture your mind, body, and spirit, reminding yourself of the lessons learned and the growth yet to come.

In moments of doubt or impatience, think of the bamboo. Let it serve as a beacon of hope and a testament to the profound growth that often remains unseen until its moment arrives. Believe in the power of persistence, in the beauty of patience, and most importantly, in the magic that lies within you.

As you step into the world, equipped with the wisdom and insights from our journey together, remember that growth is a lifelong endeavor. The pages of "Happy New You!" may have ended, but your story is still being written, with every challenge faced, every lesson learned, and every dream chased.

Keep growing. Keep evolving. And always remember, every step you take, no matter how small, is a step towards a brighter, happier, and newer you. The bamboo waited five years for its moment of glory, and when it arrived, it was spectacular. Yours is coming too. So, nurture yourself, believe in the journey, and embrace the beautiful uncertainty of the future.

Thank you for walking this path with me. May the spirit of the bamboo guide you, reminding you of the strength that lies beneath the surface, and the boundless potential that awaits.

Stay on course, revisit these pages whenever you need, and always, always remember: Your best days are still ahead.

A Heartfelt Thank You

As the author of this book, I want to express my deepest gratitude to you for choosing "Happy New You." I am honored and humbled to have shared these principles with you. My greatest joy lies in knowing that these pages have ignited the spark of transformation in your life.

Your commitment to your personal growth and dedication to implementing these habits have inspired me, and I am immensely proud of you. Your willingness to embrace change and take steps towards a better version of yourself is commendable.

Share Your Successes

I would love to hear your stories of triumph, your moments of growth, and the incredible changes you've experienced over the course of a year. Please feel free to share your success stories with me; you can reach me through my website, email, or social media platforms. Your stories will not only inspire me but also have the potential to inspire others on their journey to a Happy New You.

Beyond This Book

As you reflect on your year of growth and transformation, remember that "Happy New You" is merely a starting point—a launching pad for continuous improvement. Embrace the wisdom you've gained and let it guide you in the years to come.

The principles you've learned here are not limited to a single year; they are tools to carry with you throughout your lifetime. As you encounter new challenges and opportunities, remember the lessons you've embraced—cultivate gratitude, conquer procrastination, and embrace change fearlessly.

A Life of Happy New Years

With the principles of Happy New You as your foundation, you have the power to create a life of joy, purpose, and fulfillment— not just for one year, but for all the years to come. The journey of growth never ends, and every day presents a new canvas for you to paint the life you desire.

As you continue to celebrate your Happy New You, know that you hold the key to a life of boundless possibilities. May your heart be filled with gratitude for the person you've become and the limitless potential within you.

Closing Thoughts

As we come to the end of "Happy New You—52 Habits to Creating The Life You Want," I want to once again thank you for being a part of this journey. May you continue to walk the path of self-discovery, empowerment, and growth, creating Happy New Years year after year.

With love, gratitude, and the belief in your infinite potential,

Dr. Wendy

GOALS/THOUGHTS

SUGGESTED READING

'Comfort Crisis,' by Michael Easter

'Sugar Impact Diet,' by JJ Virgin

'Bulletproof Diet,' by Dave Asprey

'The Candida Cure,' by Ann Boroch

'5 Second Rule,' by Mel Robbins

'Lazy F*cks Don't Live to 100', by Tom Broadwell

'The Power of Habit,' by Charles Duhigg

'Self Mastery,' by Bogdan Juncewicz

'Miracle Morning,' by Hal Elrod

'Atomic Habits,' by James Clear

'The Body Keeps The Score,' by Bessel van der Kolk, MD

'Complete Guide To Fasting,' by Jason Fung

REFERENCES

Chapter 3

Dr. Jack W. Shields, M.D., Lymph, lymph glands, and homeostasis. Lymphology, v25, n4, Dec. 1992, p. 147

Ma, Yue, et al. The Effect of Diaphragmatic Breathing on Attention, Negative Affect and Stress in Healthy Adults. Psychol, 2017 Jun 6.

Zaccaro, et al. How Breath-Control Can Change Your Life: A Systematic Review on Psycho-Physiological Correlates of Slow Breathing. Front Hum Neurosci, 2018; 12: 353.

Chapter 4

Zhang, Du, et al. Effects of Dehydration and Rehydration on Cognitive Performance and Mood among Male College Students in Cangzhou, China: A Self-Controlled Trial. Int J Environ Res Public Health, 2019 Jun; 16(11): 1891.

Judge, Bellar, et al. Hydration to Maximize Performance and Recovery: Knowledge, Attitudes, and Behaviors Among Collegiate Track and Field Throwers. J Hum Kinet. 2021 Jul; 79: 111-122.

Arca, K., Singh, R., Dehydration and Headache. Curr Pain Headache Rep, 2021; 25(8): 56.

Ok, Soo-Minn, et al. Dehydration as an Etiologic Factor of Halitosis: A Case Control Study. J Oral Med Pain, 2021;46:117-124.

Fox, Alice J. Sophia, MSc, et al. The Basic Science of Articular Cartilage. Sports Health. 2009 Nov; 1(6): 461-468.

Chapter 5

Nedeltcheva, et al. Insufficient sleep undermines dietary efforts to reduce adiposity. Annals Internal Medicine, 2010 Oct 5: 153(7):435-441

Besedovsky, L., Lange, T., & Born, J. (2012). Sleep and immune function. Pflugers Archiv : European journal of physiology, 463(1), 121-137.

Pack, A. I., Pack, A. M., Rodgman, E., Cucchiara, A., Dinges, D. F., & Schwab, C. W. (1995). Characteristics of crashes attributed to the driver having fallen asleep. *Accident Analysis & Prevention*, 27(6), 769-775.

Chapter 6

Blades, R. Protecting the Brain from Bad News. CMAJ, 2021 Mar 22; 193(12): E428-E429.

Yang, et al. The effect of mindfulness intervention on internet negative news perception and processing: An implicit and explicit approach. Front Psychol, 2023; 14: 1071078.

Chapter 7

Sanaz Fasihi, et al. Effect of Alkaline Drinking Water on Bone Density of Postmenopausal Women with Osteoporosis. J Menopausal Med 2021 Aug; 27(2): 94-101.

Chapter 8

Stamatakis, et al. Association of wearable device-measured vigorous intermittent lifestyle physical activity with mortality. Nature Medicine, volume 28, pages 2521-2529 (2022).

Chapter 9

Monda, et al. Exercise Modifies the Gut Microbiota with Positive Health Effects. Oxid Med Cell Longev, 2017; 2017: 3831972.

Kuttner, et al. A randomized trial of yoga for adolescents with irritable bowel syndrome. Pain Res Manage, 2006 Winter; 11(4): 217-224.

Chapter 10

Buresh and Giller. Integrated Nutrient Management, Soil Fertility, and Sustainable Agriculture: Current Issues and Future Challenges. Journal Nutrient Cycling in Agroecosystems in 1998.

Davis, Donald R. Changes in USDA Food Composition Data for 43 Garden Crops, 1950 to 1999". Journal of the American College of Nutrition in 2004.

Martineau AR, Jolliffe DA, Hooper RL, et al. Vitamin D supplementation to prevent acute respiratory tract infections: systematic review and meta-analysis of individual participant data. JAMA. 2017;317(4):375-381.

Chapter 11

Trasmundi, et al. How Readers Beget Imagining. Front Psychol, 2020; 11: 531682.

Chapter 12

Feland, et al. The Effect of Duration of Stretching of the Hamstring Muscle Group for Increasing Range of Motion in

People Aged 65 Years or Older. Physical Therapy, Volume 81, Issue 5, 1 May 2001, Pages 1110-1117.

Chapter 13

Ferguson, et al. Effectiveness of wearable activity trackers to increase physical activity and improve health: a systematic review of systematic reviews and meta-analyses. Lancet Digital Health 2022,4:e615-26.

Chapter 14

Mead, M. Nathaniel. Benefits of Sunlight: A Bright Spot for Human Health. Environ Health Perspect, 2008 Apr; 116(4): A160-A167.

Alfredsson, et al. Insufficient Sun Exposure Has Become a Real Public Health Problem.

Int J Environ Res Public Health, 2020 Jul; 17(14): 5014.

Kent, Shia T, et al. Effect of Sunlight Exposure on Cognitive Function Among Depressed and Non Depressed Participants: a REGARDS cross-sectional study. Environ Health. 2009, July; 8:34.

Chapter 15

Oschman, Chevalier, Brown. The effects of grounding (earthing) on inflammation, the immune response, wound healing, and prevention and treatment of chronic inflammatory and autoimmune disease. J Inflamm Res 2015; 8: 83-96.

Sinatra, et al. Grounding-The universal anti-inflammatory remedy. Biomed J 2023 Feb; 46(1): 11-16

Chapter 16

Wooden, John. https://www.thewoodeneffect.com/pyramid-of-success/

Chapter 17

Archila, et al. Simple Bodyweight Training Improves Cardiorespiratory Fitness with Minimal Time Commitment: A Contemporary Application of the 5BX Approach. Int J Exerc Sci. 2021; 14(3): 93-100.

Kline, Christopher. The bidirectional relationship between exercise and sleep: Implications for exercise adherence and sleep improvement. Am J Lifestyle Med. 2014 Nov-Dec; 8(6): 375-379.

Chapter 18

Baldridge, Rebecca. The Rule of 72: How It Works And Why It Matters.

Forbes Magazine, April 10, 2023.

Chapter 19

Clason, George. The Richest Man in Babylon. 1926.

Chapter 20

Vairo, et al. Systematic Review of Efficacy for Manual Lymphatic Drainage Techniques in Sports Medicine and Rehabilitation: An Evidence-Based Practice Approach. J Manip Ther. 2009; 17(3): e80-e89.

Meier, et al. Standardized massage interventions as protocols for the induction of psychophysiological relaxation in the laboratory: a block randomized, controlled trial. Scientific Reports, 2020; 10 (1)

University of Konstanz. Ten minutes of massage or rest will help your body fight stress. ScienceDaily, 18 September 2020.

Chapter 21

Gevers-Montoro, et al. Clinical Effectiveness and Efficacy of Chiropractic Spinal Manipulation for Spine Pain. Front Pain Res (Lausanne), 2021; 2: 765921.

Ogura, et al. Cerebral metabolic changes in men after chiropractic spinal manipulation for neck pain. Altern Ther Health Med. 2011 Nov-Dec;17(6):12-7.

Acharya M, Chopra D, Smith AM, Fritz JM, Martin BC. Associations Between Early Chiropractic Care and Physical Therapy on Subsequent Opioid Use Among Persons With Low Back Pain in Arkansas. Journal of Chiropractic Medicine. 2022 May 21.

Trager RJ, Daniels CJ, Perez JA, Casselberry RM, Dusek JA. Association between chiropractic spinal manipulation and lumbar discectomy in adults with lumbar disc herniation and radiculopathy: retrospective cohort study using United States' data. BMJ Open. 2022 Dec 1;12(12):e068262.

Chapter 22

Gizem Kivrak, et al. Effects of electromagnetic fields exposure on the antioxidant defense system. J Microsc Ultrastruct 2017 Oct-Dec; 5(4): 167-176.

Chapter 23

Otake, Keiko. People become happier through kindness: A counting kindnesses intervention. J Happiness Stud. 2006 Sep; 7(3): 361-375.

Cregg, et al. Healing through helping: an experimental investigation of kindness, social activities, and reappraisal as well-being interventions, The Journal of Positive Psychology, 12 Dec 2022.

Kumar, A., & Epley, N. A little good goes an unexpectedly long way: Underestimating the positive impact of kindness on recipients. *Journal of Experimental Psychology: General, 152(1),* 236-252.

Chapter 24

van Oyen Witvliet, et al. Granting Forgiveness or Harboring Grudges: Implications for Emotion, Physiology, and Health. Psychological Science, Vol. 12, No. 2 (Mar., 2001), pp. 117-123 (7 pages)

Toussaint, et al. Forgiveness, Stress, and Health: a 5-Week Dynamic Parallel Process Study. Ann Behav Med. 2016 Oct;50(5):727-735

Chapter 26

Michalski, et al. Relationship between sense of community belonging and self-rated health across life stages. SSM Popul Health 2020 Dec; 12: 100676.

Chapter 27

Ames, et al. Interpersonal assertiveness: Inside the balancing act. Social and Personality Psychology Compass, June 2017, Volume 11, Issue 6, e12317.

Koutsimani, et al. The Relationship Between Burnout, Depression, and Anxiety: A Systematic Review and Meta-Analysis. Front Psychol. 2019; 10: 284.

Urban, Melissa. The Book Of Boundaries - Set the Limits That Will Set You Free. October 2022

Cloud, Henry, and John Townsend. Boundaries. October 2017.

Chapter 28

Becker, Joshua. The Minimalist Home. December 2018

Sasaki, Fumio. Goodbye, things. April 2017

Chapter 29

House, et al. Social relationships and health. Science. 1988 Jul 29;241(4865):540-5.

Martino, et al. The Connection Prescription: Using the Power of Social Interactions and the Deep Desire for Connectedness to Empower Health and Wellness. Am J Lifestyle Med 2015 Oct 7;11(6):466-475. eCollection 2017 Nov-Dec.

Chapter 30

Tasler, Nick. Just Make a Decision Already. Harvard Business Review. October 2013.

Chapter 31

Carnegie, Dale. How to Win Friends and Influence People. November 1936.

Schafer, Jack, et al. The Like Switch. January 2015

Fox Cabane, Olivia. The Charisma Myth. March 2013

Chapter 32

Johnson, Ph.D., John A. The Psychology of Expectations. Why unrealistic expectations are premeditated resentments. Psychology Today. February 2018.

Chapter 33

Berk, LS, et al. Neuroendocrine and stress hormone changes during mirthful laughter. Am J Med Sci. 1989 Dec;298(6):390-6.

Yim, JongEun. Therapeutic Benefits of Laughter in Mental Health: A Theoretical Review. Tohoku J Exp Med. 2016 Jul;239(3):243-9.

Chapter 34

Watkins, P. C., et al. Gratitude and subjective well-being: Cultivating gratitude for a harvest of happiness. In *Research anthology on rehabilitation practices and therapy: Concepts, methodologies, tools, and applications* (pp. 1737-1759). 2021.

Chapter 35

Stahl, James E., et al. Relaxation Response and Resiliency Training and Its Effect on Healthcare Resource Utilization. Plos One. October 13, 2015.

Toussaint, Loren, et al. Effectiveness of Progressive Muscle Relaxation, Deep Breathing, and Guided Imagery in Promoting Psychological and Physiological States of Relaxation. Evid Based Complement Alternat Med 2021; 2021: 5924040.

Chapter 36

Ussery, Emily, et al. Joint Prevalence of Sitting Time and Leisure-Time Physical Activity Among US Adults- 2015-2016. JAMA. 2018;320(19):2036-2038.

Chandler, Meredith. Sitting Disease: The Terrifying Facts of Prolonged Sitting. Ergonomics Health Association. January 2020.

Biswas, Aviroop, et al. Sedentary time and its association with risk for disease incidence, mortality, and hospitalization in adults: a systematic review and meta-analysis. Ann Intern Med. 2015 Jan 20;162(2):123-32.

Chapter 37

Bohannon, Richard. Hand-grip dynamometry predicts future outcomes in aging adults. J Geriatr Phys Ther. 2008;31(1):3-10.

Mendelow, et al. Lumbar disc disease: the effect of inversion on clinical symptoms and a comparison of the rate of surgery after inversion therapy with the rate of surgery in neurosurgery controls. Journal of Physical Therapy Science. Volume 33, Issue 11, 2021.

Chapter 38

Tan, et al. Being Creative Makes You Happier: The Positive Effect of Creativity on Subjective Well-Being. Int J Environ Res Public Health, 2021 Jul; 18(14): 7244.

Suttie, Jill. Doing Something Creative Can Boost Your Well-Being. Berkeley.edu. March 2017.

Chapter 39

Shatte, et al. The Positive Effect of Resilience on Stress and Business Outcomes in Difficult Work Environments. Journal of Occupational and Environmental Medicine, 59(2):p 135-140, February 2017.

Bonanno, George. Loss, trauma, and human resilience: have we underestimated the human capacity to thrive after extremely aversive events? Am Psychol. 2004 Jan;59(1):20-8.

Chapter 40

Batts Allen, Ashley, Leary Mark R. Self-Compassion, Stress, and Coping. Soc Personal Psychol Compass. 2010 Feb 1; 4(2): 107-118.

Smith, Jennifer L. Self-compassion and resilience in senior living residents. Seniors Housing and Care Journal 23.1 (2015): 17-31.

Chapter 41

McRaven, Admiral William H. Make Your Bed: Little Things That Can Change Your Life... And Maybe The World. April 2017.

Chapter 42

Blackwell, Simon E, et al. Optimism and mental imagery: A possible cognitive marker to promote well- being? Psychiatry Res 2013 Mar 30; 206(1): 56–61.

Cheema, Amar/Bagchi, Rajesh. The Effect of Goal Visualization on Goal Pursuit : Implications for Individuals and Managers. SSRN 2011.

Byers, Taylor. The Power of the Mind Through Visualization. Swimming World. May 2022.

Chapter 43

Monae, Athalia. 6 Things You Gain By Embracing Failure and Learning From Mistakes. Entrepreneur, MAR 23, 2023.

Chapter 45

Eby, Lillian T, et al. Does Mentoring Matter? A Multidisciplinary Meta-Analysis Comparing Mentored and Non-Mentored Individuals. J Vocal Behav. 2008 Apr; 72(2): 254-267.

Chapter 46

Robbins, Mel. The 5 Second Rule: Transform your Life, Work, and Confidence with Everyday Courage. February 28, 2017.

Chapter 47

Newman, Kira M. Four Reasons to Cultivate Patience- Good things really do come to those who wait. Greater Good Magazine. April 4, 2016.

Chapter 48

Anton, Barry S., PhD. APA President. Embracing Change. American Psychological Association. January 2015, Vol 46, No. 1

Chapter 49

Riess, Helen, MD. The Science of Empathy. J Patient Exp. 2017 Jun; 4(2): 74-77.

Abramson, Ashley. Cultivating empathy: Psychologists' research offers insight into why it's so important to practice the "right" kind of empathy, and how to grow these skills: American Psychological Association. November 1, 2021. Vol. 52 No. 8.

Chapter 50

Benjamin Harkin, et al. **Does Monitoring Goal Progress Promote Goal Attainment? A Meta-Analysis of the Experimental Evidence.** *Psychological Bulletin*, 2015.

Chapter 51

Zenger, Jack. Taking Responsibility Is The Highest Mark Of Great Leaders. Forbes. July 16, 2015.

Coleman, John. Take Ownership of Your Actions by Taking Responsibility. Harvard Business Review. Aug 30, 2012

ABOUT THE AUTHOR

Dr. Wendy Schauer, DC, RKC, is an esteemed chiropractor and wellness innovator with over thirty years of dedicated service, passionately guiding individuals toward peak health and empowerment. As the founder of Community Chiropractic, P.S., and the creative force behind Abundant Fitness Center, Inc., she stands out as the first female chiropractor to achieve the Russian Kettlebell Certification, integrating this expertise into a holistic approach that benefits body, mind, and spirit. Her commitment to personalized, innovative care and her pioneering work in chiropractic pediatrics and Ehlers-Danlos Syndrome support her belief in healing as a bespoke journey for each individual.

With her new book, "Happy New You!", Dr. Schauer offers a vibrant, transformative roadmap that serves as a life atlas, inviting readers to embark on a journey toward personal renewal and vibrant health. This work builds on the foundation of her acclaimed previous book, "The 7 Steps to Amazing Health!", extending her vision of empowering individuals to navigate their wellness paths with confidence and clarity. Her accolades, including the YWCA Women of Achievement Award, reflect her profound impact on community health and her unwavering dedication to fostering resilience and self-empowerment, making her a beacon of inspiration in the wellness world.

Made in United States
Troutdale, OR
11/08/2024

24560226R00164